EBURY PRESS

YOGIPLATE

Radhavallabha Das is an acclaimed chef, author, former monk, yoga teacher, speaker and life coach. He has over two decades of experience in sāttvic and Ayurvedic vegetarian cooking, developed by reading Ayurvedic texts. He is the founder of Yogi Plate, an organization dedicated to educating people about sāttvic cooking.

After completing his MTech from IIT, he decided to become a monk at ISKCON, Mumbai, to dedicate his life to the service of society. There he cooked for 250 residents of the ashram daily for more than a decade. As head chef, he led a team of highly acclaimed chefs who were featured in National Geographic Channel's *India's Megakitchens* series, serving about 10,000 plates of sāttvic food every day. He was also the cook of his Gurudev, HH Radhanath Swami, for seventeen years.

But the love for Ayurveda grew from discussions with Dr Sanjay Pisharodi, a fellow ashram resident with an MBBS degree and also great knowledge of Ayurveda. Radhavallabha Das has conducted more than 200 cooking workshops across the world and has held seminars on the importance of an Ayurvedic diet, including at the headquarters of Microsoft, Amazon and Intel in the USA.

Currently he lives with his wife Hansapriya in Silicon Valley in California. He is working with a team to bring healthy food to people through cloud kitchens, live cooking workshops, seminars and one-on-one consulting.

yogiplate

The FUNDAMENTALS *of* SĀTTVIC FOOD

Radhavallabha Das

Foreword by GAURANGA DAS,
author of *The Art of Resilience*

EBURY
PRESS

An imprint of Penguin Random House

EBURY PRESS

USA | Canada | UK | Ireland | Australia
New Zealand | India | South Africa | China

Ebury Press is part of the Penguin Random House group of companies
whose addresses can be found at global.penguinrandomhouse.com

Published by Penguin Random House India Pvt. Ltd
4th Floor, Capital Tower 1, MG Road,
Gurugram 122 002, Haryana, India

Penguin
Random House
India

First published in Ebury Press by Penguin Random House India 2021

10 9 8 7 6 5 4 3 2

The views and opinions expressed in this book are the author's own and the facts are as reported by him which have been verified to the extent possible, and the publishers are not in any way liable for the same.

The book is designed to provide helpful information on the subjects discussed. This book is not meant to be used, nor should it be used, to diagnose or treat any medical condition. For diagnosis or treatment of any medical problem, consult your physician. The publisher and author are not responsible for any specific health or allergy needs that may require medical supervision and are not liable for any damages or negative consequences from any treatment, action, application or preparation, to any person reading or following the information in this book.

ISBN 9780143454533

Typeset in Adobe Caslon Pro by Manipal Technologies Limited, Manipal
Printed at Manipal Technologies Limited, India

www.penguin.co.in

FSC
www.fsc.org
MIX
Paper from responsible sources
FSC® C043100

To my mother: Madhuri Pattanayak
(who nourished me with a sāttvic diet all my childhood)

and

To my dear friend: Dr Sanjay Pisharodi
(who impressed the concepts of
Ayurvedic diet in my heart very deeply)

Contents

Foreword

I am thrilled to learn about *Yogiplate.* I see this as not just a deeply researched writing but a revelation from the core of Radhavallabha Das's heart, nurtured over decades.

My association with Radhavallabha Das dates back to the 1990s and since then, we have had many cherished moments together at the monastery in Chowpatty, Mumbai. Apt to the context of this book, most of those moments were nourished in the aromatic kitchen of the temple or in the famed yatra kitchens that we erected during the annual pilgrimage to holy places in India. Radhavallabha Das is passionate about cooking. But, beyond that, he is so mindful about the finer nuances of cooking that he strived to deliver a fine dining experience not just for the hungry belly but for the yearning soul as well.

Tasting food is a divine activity of directly experiencing God's inconceivable creation. The diversity in the types of food made available seasonally, topographically and nutritionally is something that has left scientists awestruck since centuries. However, based on numerous reports produced by the United Nations and the Food and Drug Administration (FDA), there are heart-wrenching numbers on food waste. Global food waste could feed 2 billion people a year and creates 3.6 billion tons of carbon dioxide-equivalent greenhouse gas.

Further, 28 per cent of the world's agricultural area is used to produce wasted food. Radhavallabha Das worked diligently to formulate hundreds of recipes into Excel sheets and prevented food loss while scaling up the production, notably so during large-scale cooking. He has applied all his technical education to cooking to achieve this. This book will educate readers about the material and spiritual value of food and thus inspire them to be more conscious of the optimal utilization of food.

The Chāndogya Upaniṣad says, '*Āhāra-śuddhau sattva-śuddhiḥ sattva-śuddhau dhruvā smṛtiḥ smṛti-lambhe sarva-granthīnāṁ vipramokṣaḥ.*' When one's eatables become sanctified, and by eating sanctified foodstuffs, one's very existence becomes purified; by the purification of existence, finer tissues in the memory become sanctified, and when memory is sanctified, one can think of the path of liberation. With this foundational principle, together we cooked tons of sāttvic food that has touched the hearts of thousands of people. Radhavallabha Das visited many ancient Vedic temples, studying their traditional cooking under the guidance of experienced cooks. In *Yogiplate*, he draws inspiration from the annals of Ayurvedic texts to delve deep into the value quotient offered by different food items, the wellness element associated with each and the personalized food recommendations based on one's unique body type to nourish a sound body, serene mind and spirited soul.

To sum up: through the book, this yogi serves on a plate the science of Ayurveda and the reader can have a delectable experience by experimenting with this science through the yoga of sāttvic cooking and mindful living.

3 July 2021 Gauranga Das,

Govardhan Eco Village, near Mumbai

Prologue

I became interested in Ayurveda when I learnt how the concepts of *vāta*, *pitta* and *kapha* are used to identify each person's unique character, including eating habits. It's now been more than twenty years since I first learnt about them. Like many of you, I too have scanned the Internet to learn how to cook and eat things that suit me best, but many seemingly contradictory pieces of information only confused me.

I am a certified yoga teacher from Shivananda Yoga Peetham, and as a monk, I have cooked *sāttvic* food for more than two decades in the monastery of ISKCON Chowpatty in Mumbai. The sheer sāttvic cooking experience (sometimes over 10,000 plates in a day) pushed me to conduct hundreds of sāttvic cooking workshops along with yoga and talks on Ayurvedic diet and lifestyle. I did this repeatedly across many countries, including India, the US and many in Europe. These workshops shaped my understanding of Ayurveda and inspired me to teach and write on the importance of sāttvic Ayurvedic cooking. I am confident that this lifestyle book will help one and all.

For this purpose, when I delved a little deeper into Ayurvedic cooking, I realized it's not as simple as saying you shouldn't eat kheer and yoghurt at the same time, or tamarind is bad for you. It depends on a lot of factors that are unique to each person. I sensed the need for a book that could simply help you learn and practise the tenets of Ayurveda to make sure you eat what is best *for you.* So, I consulted experienced Ayurvedic doctors and studied age-old traditions. My objective is to clarify all the confusing and contradictory things you might have read or heard about Ayurvedic principles of cooking and eating and help you design your individual food profile.

For instance, some acclaimed doctors say that you shouldn't have bananas and milk together as this combination will create toxins in the digestive tract due to indigestion. But all my childhood, I have seen this combination being offered to idols of Lord Shiva. But then I read another article in which an Ayurvedic doctor had explained that consuming milk and banana together is fine unless a person has a predisposition to kapha and obesity and is prone to cough and cold. The *Caraka-Saṃhitā* in Sutra Sthana delineates that two food ingredients with a similar nature can be combined. As both milk and banana are sweet in nature, it is fine to consume them together as long as it suits your body. On the other hand, these items are heavy to digest individually and combining them makes it even more challenging for the body to digest unless your digestive fire is high. But how do you determine that? The answer is: by understanding what kind of body type you have. We will study these things in detail in the later chapters of this book but for now, let's just say if you have a high metabolism and struggle to put on weight, a banana milkshake will suit you well. For those who tend to get bloated or feel heavy after eating rich food, it is best avoided.

Nevertheless, the world we live in today has moved far away from an Ayurvedic way of living, though the principles still hold true. More complications arise when bananas that are artificially ripened using carbides are consumed with chilled, pasteurized milk. The bananas that are available tend to be slightly sour (owing to artificial ripening). And since milk does not go well with any sour food, this combination should not be had by anyone unless they are sure of the quality of the ingredients.

Usually, most people look to change their diet when they are ill, have a deficiency or want to achieve a specific goal such as losing weight. Modern medicine tries to treat sick people but has no solutions to keep healthy people healthy. On the other hand, the guiding principle in Ayurveda is that all who practise it lead a long and healthy life. It discusses in detail how to prevent diseases. It recognizes that the stomach is the birthplace of all illnesses. Thus, by eating healthy, one can potentially protect oneself against all diseases. Modern medicine has started acknowledging this but still has a long way to go.

So, pondering over all these topics, when I sat down to write this book, I decided to put together all the Ayurvedic principles specific to diet—and eating according to your body type—in a simple manner. Years of study in science and technology made me believe that life follows simple linear rules that can be translated into a mathematical equation. This propelled me to try to create a master table or equation that considers all the factors related to various ingredients and helps one evaluate their food profile. But life is much more than a mathematical equation, and I truly thank God for that. It's not as simple as saying A+B will lead to a result C.

Numerous factors determine which food will suit you and which will not. Some of them are as abstract as the colour of the clothes you wear. Because different colours absorb different radiations and alter our body temperature—and effectively, the strength of our digestive fire differently.

Substances found in nature can be present with all kinds of contradictory combinations of properties too. For example, cilantro and coconut water are both cooling and igniting. Thus, it becomes hard to incorporate it all into one linear equation. As I wrote, I gradually realized that there are so many things people deserve to know. So, instead of formulating an equation, I tried to arrive at the perfect, balanced plate of food for you—the Yogi Plate.

How do you build this perfect plate? For this, we need to know our own nature based on the principles of kapha, pitta and vāta, as well as the nature of food. This book will guide you in both aspects. Then you can conclude what food is good for you and what isn't. That will be the first step to building a happy, healthy life.

We need to appreciate that an ingredient can't always be categorized into just one box and its nature often overlaps with that of other ingredients. Each substance is a unique mixture of the five elements of the universe. As a result, each substance interacts in a particular way with the human body. Not all of it is still completely understood and we can only marvel at the complexity of nature and the creations of God. Thus, certain substances can exhibit properties and effects that are entirely contradictory. There is always a general pattern and also the exception. We may initially study the characteristics of each ingredient separately, but we will also learn which ingredients they can combine with so that they balance and stabilize each other. After all, how we combine them with each other also impacts our health. Even the way food is cooked, served, stored, etc. determines whether the food will nurture us or cause discomfort.

This book tries to inculcate simple, pure Vedic traditions so that we can eat well and also avoid the side effects of a modern lifestyle.

Throughout the book, we will delve into the concept of digestion as Ayurveda describes it. Proper digestion prevents food from degenerating into harmful substances, which tend to cause various diseases, from a nagging backache to a chronic condition, such as diabetes. Thus, digestion is the main focus of a perfect Ayurvedic meal. All other factors, such as choosing the ingredients or spice, are dependent on digestion.

We will also examine different body types and the characteristics of some common ingredients—all of this together will help you choose the food that suits your body.

Another important aspect that we will discuss is the connection between mind and sāttvic diet. Sāttvic food builds a lot of positivity, which is pivotal to robust mental health. We will see how food cooked with a caring attitude nourishes our mind and how the ingredients used affect it.

This book is not just for those who want to follow a yogic lifestyle. Once you understand how your food is digested and how the body reacts to it, you'll be inspired to keep eating and cooking according to the Ayurvedic principles. This book will be helpful for young parents taking care of growing kids while trying to keep themselves healthy. Those trying to understand the diet dynamics while working under stress will also gather some effective solutions from this book. Young kids and youths need to understand these principles to safeguard themselves from sicknesses and the practice will protect them from their mid-age health crisis. Having seen the positive results, I follow all of these principles for my own diet.

As for myself, I was born and raised in a Vaishnava family, and while I was in school and lived with my family, I ate only sāttvic food. I remember my mother cooking restaurant-style food at home to discourage us from eating out. But when I left home for higher education, I started experimenting with different food, including non-vegetarian food. However, after seeing a chicken getting slaughtered, I decided to stay vegetarian. Later, I became a monk and lived in an ashram for over twenty years. I continue to follow a sāttvic diet till today. In these years, my happy and steady service has been cooking. I cooked for my spiritual master and other monks at the ashram. Every year, I had the opportunity to head a team of cooks to prepare meals for large gatherings of pilgrims at Vrindavan, Mayapur and many other holy places. We would pack up the kitchen in trucks and travel to these places and set up the kitchen in agricultural fields. Popularly known as 'The Yatra Kitchen', one of these kitchens was featured in National Geographic Channel's *India's Megakitchens* documentary series.

As my cooking adventures continued, I studied Vedic literature and was amazed to learn how much it is about food. I visited several ancient Vedic temples where the culture of sāttvic cooking still exists and was surprised to see how each preparation was cooked, following the Ayurvedic principles. I also travelled to Italy to learn Italian cuisine, especially the art of baking traditional pizzas in wood-fired ovens. Later, I helped in setting up pizzerias in two Hare Krishna temples. During my visits to south-east Asian countries, I learnt a lot about their traditional cuisines that have become internationally popular. I studied various Ayurvedic books like *Astānga Hṛdayam* (Sutra Sthana), *Bhojanakutuhalam*, etc., that specifically spoke of healthy dietary practices for healthy people. The main purpose of cooking is to care for and nourish the body and mind of the consumers. All these studies were crucial to this end. All these experiences have helped me write this book.

I never planned to be a chef in my life. But I had a passion for the kitchen. So, when I look back, I feel a deep and sublime sense of satisfaction. I am grateful to all those who inspired this passion in me and opened up opportunities to fulfil that passion. Through my service, I have realized that each of us deserves to live long, healthy lives. This book will help you design a diet that imparts health and vitality.

Section One

Know Thyself: Understanding Our Nature

Tridoṣa: The Three Building Blocks
Determining Our Tridoṣic Nature or Prakṛti
Classification of Tridoṣic Nature
Sātmya: Acquired Nature
Triguṇa: Understanding Your Personality
Classifications of Triguṇa Nature

Know Thyself: Understanding Our Nature

'Be yourself . . . the world will adjust.'

—*Germany Kent*

The world today has become like a superconductor, where not only is information transfer happening at lightning speed but also produce of all kinds is being shipped overnight. Just walk into a well-stocked store and you will find an array of all types of food throughout the year. As a result, it has become increasingly confusing to trace which food is local or which is seasonal.

Food is a very sophisticated fuel and needs to be considered carefully before being consumed. Just like a car engine that runs on petrol cannot run on diesel, we should not consume food that is not wholly natural and cannot be digested by our bodies.

Growing up in a small town in the state of Odisha in India, I remember, as the youngest child of the family, how fussy I was about my food choices. My choices were quite different from those of my siblings, and that forced my mother to prepare my meals separately.

Ayurveda, which deals with life span (Āyu means life span or longevity and Veda means knowledge), explains that each human being is unique and so is the quality and quantity of their diet. As we study Ayurvedic literature, it becomes more evident that one man's food may be poison for another. Similarly, eating the same type of factory-processed food without understanding our design can potentially cause many health issues. Eating processed food once in a while is okay but habitual consumption can cause harm that will gradually build up to an irreparable state. A lot of research points to how diet is connected to many modern-day sicknesses. The number of people who suffer from certain chronic diseases—such as bronchitis, asthma, diabetes, etc.—has increased dramatically in the last few decades.

Therefore, Ayurveda stresses that our diet should be according to the design or nature of our individual bodies. It is not the body that adjusts to the food. If the nature of the food is in harmony with the nature of our body, it will be efficiently processed by the digestive system. So, to understand the correct diet for yourself, it is important to understand the following:

1. The nature of the person
2. The nature of food

Modern lifestyles have often taken us away from ourselves. We simply try to 'become' something or someone and, in the process, forget who we are. The 'reel world' has gained more significance in our lives than the 'real world'. If we do not know who we are or what our real nature is, how can we remain happy and healthy? Whom should we nourish? Our dreams or our true selves? Yet, we hardly ever make an effort to understand our true nature. Understanding our nature not only helps improve our diet but also helps us know what activities are suitable for us and what our dreams and aspirations are. The goal of this book is to help you understand your nature, the nature of various food ingredients (uncooked and cooked) and then map both to design a food profile that nourishes and maintains that nature.

Ayurveda uses two fundamental concepts to understand a person's nature or *prakṛti* (as termed in Sanskrit):

1. Tri-doṣa or the three 'building blocks' that can sustain as well as damage life forms.
2. Tri-guṇa or the three 'modes/types' of nature that develop our personality.

Triguṇas influence our psyche, which shapes our behavioural traits, while tridoṣa is generally responsible for the physical characteristics. Tridoṣa builds and helps the functioning of a healthy, strong body, whereas triguṇa influences our likes and dislikes. So, in a sense, tridoṣa is responsible for the hardware (the body) while triguṇa is responsible for the software (the mind). All of these play an important role in designing our diet, which is a major source of our nourishment.

Tri-doṣa: The Three Building Blocks

The same calm and peaceful ocean that helps ships sail smoothly to their destination can destroy and drown them in moments when it goes out of balance due to the agitation caused by a fiery sun and rising wind.

Let's try to understand the tridoṣa, the building blocks. The Sanskrit word *tri* means three and the word *doṣa* means faults. Yes, the three building blocks are termed faulty. *Duṣyanti iti doṣa:* to be more precise, the impact is faulty. It is strange, but what sustains our material body can also kill it. Now, one may ask why the faulty (killing) side of these building blocks and not the sustaining quality is the essence. It is called tridoṣa or three faults instead of *tristhiti* or three sustainers because ultimately, these building blocks are successful as destroyers of the body rather than sustaining it. It is not a pessimistic view, my dear readers. Rather, it is an indicator of reality to warn us how much care we need to take to keep our bodies and minds healthy. When these doṣas are in balance, we relish good health, but when the doṣas are agitated and go out of balance, they start destroying the body.

One may wonder, how can something that is destructive by nature sustain life? This is how Ācārya Vāgabhaṭa, one of the greatest Ayurvedic preceptors, describes doṣas: 'Suppose we leave a piece of bread unattended. After a day or two, some fungus will start to develop on it. Anybody who eats it will become sick as the bread has turned toxic. But after another day or two, we will observe some worms on the bread! In fact, the worms thrive on that rotting bread. How so?' Vāgabhaṭa explains that while certain combinations can sustain one form of life, they can be poisonous for another. Similarly, although kapha, pitta and vāta are poisonous in nature, in a certain balanced combination, they sustain life. **This balance is the key to good health**. The moment this balance gets disturbed, these very doṣas that build one's body will notoriously destroy it, like a rising ocean swallows up a ship. For example, imbalanced kapha produces a lot of mucus and can potentially make it tough to breathe. Imbalanced pitta causes excess heat, resulting in acidity or heartburn and is generally associated with high fever. Imbalanced vāta is the cause of pain in the body and is also known to cause restlessness.

An important aspect of diet, according to Ayurveda, is not to disturb this balance. Disturbing it is like waking up a sleeping tiger. Our diet should respect this balance while also nourishing the doṣas. So, it's important to understand the nature of our body as well as the nature of food, and accordingly match them.

What are these three faults—kapha, pitta and vāta—that Ayurveda is speaking about? It is difficult to translate each of them to a single English word as their description may need volumes. So, we will not translate the meaning and rather take them as they are and try to understand them.

Ayurveda considers that everything is made up of five basic elements, similar to what Aristotle believed. These are earth, water, air, fire and ether. These are described in Ayurveda as *pañca mahābbhūta*, meaning the five great elements. These elements combine in different ways to create tridoṣa, the building blocks of life systems (Table 1.1). The combinations are as follows:

Table 1.1: Doṣa and Material Elements

Doṣa	Elements	Quality	Function
Kapha	Earth + Water	Preserving	Anabolic
Pitta	Water + Fire	Processing	Catabolic
Vāta	Air + Space	Performing	Metabolic

Kapha combines earth and water to build the framework or the foundational structure of the body—from skin to muscles, bones and even delicate organs. It forms the foundational substance that a body needs to stand on, like moulding a statue by combining clay and water. In biochemistry, such processes are called anabolism, where complex molecules are built from simpler ones. These molecules also store energy, for example, in the form of fats. If we think of our body as a car, then all the solid framework and the auto parts of a car are kapha. So, kapha provides stability, lubrication, firmness to joints and even forbearance to withstand emotional onslaughts.

Generally, kapha is more active in the upper portion of our body, that is, the chest, neck and head. When there is an imbalance of kapha, and there is too much of it, we are primarily affected in these three areas, resulting in cold, cough, fever, etc. The imbalance also weakens the digestive system and is accompanied by a feeling of heaviness, weariness and excess sleep. When there is reduction of kapha, it causes looseness of joints, dizziness and tremors (owing to low energy). All these imbalances, when recognized in the initial stage, can be corrected by administering a proper diet. Usually, food that is earthy, wholesome and heavy is loaded with kapha. Grains, dairy, ghee and oil (such as coconut oil) have high kapha. Remember that kapha is constituted of two elements with opposing nature, viz. earth and water. Whereas earth has a fixed shape and likes not to move, water flows. Kapha is that force which brings them together to build and give shape. In that sense, kapha is neither earth nor water, but something of its own.

Pitta is more subtle. It is a combination of water and fire, which again are two elements with seemingly opposite natures. Generally, we use water to extinguish fire, so how can they co-exist together? There is a beauty about water. It takes on the quality of the element it combines with. With earth, it becomes earthy to form kapha. With fire, it becomes fiery. Water extinguishes the fire by trapping the heat. Pitta is the force that combines heat or fire with water and spreads it all over the body. From thermodynamics, we understand how water traps heat very efficiently (water's specific heat is 1 or 100 per cent, higher than any other commonly known substance).

While kapha is more active in the upper portion of our body, pitta as heat is prominently present in the stomach and thus, active in the middle portion of our body. Fire spreads out more than earth. So, pitta is more subtle and spreads out all over our body. The fire in the stomach, which is responsible for digestion, is the main seat of pitta. In a balanced state, pitta attends to digestion, vision, softness and complexion of the skin. It maintains body temperature and ignites hunger and thirst.

Through digestion, it helps break down the complex molecules of food we eat into simpler ones that the body can assimilate and use. In biochemistry, this process is known as catabolism. Just like kapha represents the framework of a car, pitta represents the fire in the engine. Just like fuel is burnt in the engine, the ingested food is digested in the stomach's fire. This fire is called *jatharāgni* in Sanskrit, literally meaning the fire (*agni*) in the stomach (*jathara*). However, digestion is much more than that. It not only derives the energy to move (the wheels of the car), but also breaks down complex molecules and absorbs them through the liver. These simple molecules provide all the raw materials for performing various tasks to preserve life and the vitality of the body. These molecules are used by kapha to form building blocks to build new cells and maintain/preserve the existing cells or combine them to store energy as fat.

Apart from digestion, pitta is also largely responsible for the health of the skin. Glowing skin is a sign of robust and balanced pitta. Imbalanced decreased pitta leads to loss of lustre, coldness and weakness in the digestive system, resulting in loss of hunger, even to the extent that we become averse to the food we love. Adversely, increased pitta can cause hunger pangs more than usual. It also makes the skin, urine, eyes and faeces appear yellow and affects sleep. Unless the digestive system is cool and sleeps, the rest of your body can't sleep.

Vāta is the subtlest of three. The closest translation of vāta could be the wind. It's a combination of air and ether. Constitutionally, vāta being dynamic pushes the air to expand and occupy the available space (ether element). But more than that, vāta—like the force that comes with the wind—

is responsible for all the movements of the body, within or without. In a car, the ignited fuel in the engine creates gases that push the pistons, which in turn rotate the gear and finally the wheels. Similarly, vāta, in its balanced state, is responsible for movements like the flow of breath, the articulation of speech, the circulation of blood, the elimination of stool and urine, perspiration, and the regulation of the immune and nervous systems. It moves the diaphragm, muscles and limbs. These activities are called metabolism in biochemistry. The energy that is created by pitta through digestion and stored by kapha is used by vāta. Without vāta, kapha and pitta are inert and lifeless. In fact, the intricate smooth functions of kapha and pitta are possible because of vāta. Balanced vāta bestows enthusiasm and vigour to perform actions and tasks of intelligence seamlessly. So, to balance vāta is very essential. But the challenge is, this doṣa is the subtlest and difficult to manage.

Vāta's primary area of operation is waist downward, although it's active throughout the body. If you don't have any joint pain or backache, just lie down flat on the floor on your back and try to slowly lift both of your legs (without bending the knees) up while inhaling. If you cannot, then your vāta is imbalanced.

Imbalanced vāta generally manifests as pain in some part of the body. We can tolerate inconvenience in kapha or pitta to a fairly high extent, but pain associated with imbalanced vāta makes one helpless and pushes us to find the cause. Ayurveda is not in favour of modern-day painkillers because they simply treat the symptoms by suppressing them. In case of pain, the nervous system, which carries the message as pain, is being suppressed. It's similar to a situation where a messenger brings us the bad news that a house is on fire and instead of putting out the fire, we subdue the messenger and pretend that everything is okay. Sometimes, the fire could have a severe cause like cancer.

Ayurveda recommends that we search for the cause of the pain or the disturbed vāta and resolve it without ignoring it. It's best if the imbalanced vāta can be resolved through diet, rest and exercise. Modern-day painkillers also cause many side effects that can affect our vital organs, such as the kidneys, heart and liver, and thus disrupt the functions of vāta further. Remember that these organs are vital because the body can't live without them. A person can continue to live without a limb, but one cannot expect to live if one of the vital organs stops functioning. So, to harm them even slightly is dangerous.

Increased vāta makes one emaciated and causes the skin to turn blackish. One experiences tremors, loss of sleep and strength, constipation, irrelevant speech, timidity and giddiness. Decreased vāta results in a debilitated body, little or no talking, low sensory perceptions and occurrence of all symptoms of increased kapha.

Another important aspect of tridoṣa is that the bones give shelter to vāta doṣa (like a solid cage), blood gives shelter to pitta and kapha resides in all the other tissues. So, imbalanced vāta causes pain in the bones and joints, imbalanced pitta affects digestive fire and skin, and imbalanced kapha chokes the channels in the tissues. One should try to bring balance to the doṣas by balancing the diet, undertaking appropriate activities and taking sufficient rest. Table 1.2 briefly features the typical qualities associated with the three doṣas.

Table 1.2: Doṣa's Attributes

Kapha	Pitta	Vāta
Heavy*	**Hot***	**Dry***
Cold	Oily	Light
Smooth	Intense	Cold
Stable	Liquid	Irregular
*** Main attributes**		

These three doṣas come together in various proportions to create different bodies, each with a unique individual nature or prakṛti.

Determining Our Tridoṣic Nature or Prakṛti

The word prakṛti has two parts: *pra* meaning 'original/prototype' and *kṛta* meaning 'creation'. Prakṛti thus means the original creation. Kapha doṣa, pitta doṣa and vāta doṣa combine to create our tridoṣic nature and bring forth the unique nature of an individual—the constitutional nature of a human being.

During conception, the tridoṣa of the sperm from the father combines with the tridoṣa of the egg from the mother to create a new tridoṣa for the baby. Now this unique tridoṣa protects the child. This combination is the child's unique signature. The combination is unique because each child's kapha, pitta and vāta constitutions are in different proportions. Ayurveda advises not to agitate or change this original creation or prakṛti.

Only expert Ayurvedic doctors can examine and understand the exact constitution of our body. They understand the imbalances, the cause of them and the remedies. Experienced doctors can determine the imbalance in the doṣas by just the touch of the pulse.

But for people like us who aren't experts, Ayurveda gives ten broad classifications to understand our basic nature.

This knowledge of our tridoṣic nature will guide us in our day-to-day actions (diet, work, sleep, exercise, sex, etc., i.e., Dinacaryā) and also how to conduct in different seasons (Ṛtucaryā). An important point to be noted in this regard is that the diet, activities, exercise and sleep are all intimately connected to each other. If we take care of one and ignore the other, then the doṣa-balance will be compromised. There are certain people who practise celibacy, or a voluntary abstinence, but they still need to regulate other aspects of their life to stay healthy. Let's learn about the different classifications so we can take a step towards being our most balanced selves.

Classification of Tridoṣic Nature

The ideal combination of these three doṣas in a person is when they are present harmoniously with equal prominence in a personality. Such people are indeed rare. Just as in a car, if the body is sturdy, the engine is powerful and the wheels move smoothly, you can drive fast for a very long distance. But if the engine and wheels are powerful but not the body, then the driver cannot afford to go fast. The engine may be able to take it but the body may collapse. For a smooth journey, the driver has to slow down. Similarly, when the doṣas are equally present, the body functions smoothly and coherently. All other doṣa combinations are considered inferior. The second-best situation is when one doṣa is prominent and the other two simply support it. But it's considered a problem if two doṣas are prominent, because then there will be a clash for prominence as the doṣas are opposite in their own constitutional nature. There can't be two leaders in one team. Such situations are delicate, and the balance can be toppled with even a little agitation. The resilience will be weaker as the inbuilt defence system is not as cooperative either. Such combinations demand more care. So, the challenge in designing an appropriate food profile in such situations becomes tougher. But in any case, whatever nature a person has acquired certainly protects that person.

In general, we fall into one of the categories as described in Chart 1.1.

Chart 1.1: Prakṛti Classification

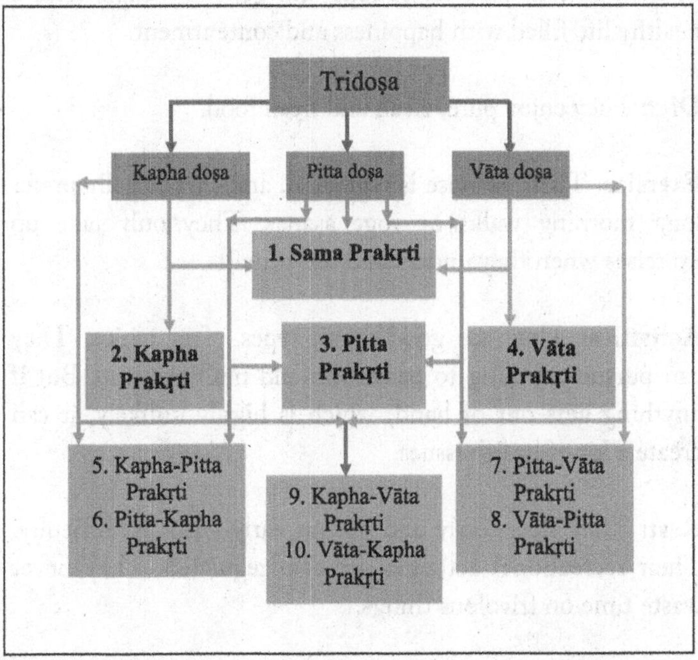

An important point to note here is that we are not discussing individual doṣas (we have already done that). Rather we are looking at the prakṛti of a person whose doṣas (one or more) have varying degrees of prominence. We will also discuss the prescribed diet-exercise-work-rest profile for each of these. This will help us to keep the doṣas in balance.

1. **Sama-Tridoṣa** (All three doṣas are equally present)

Personality: This prakṛti carrying a balanced tridoṣa (equal proportion of kapha, pitta and vāta) is the best possible constitution. These people are blessed with a balanced approach to all aspects of life. They are highly regulated in their actions and recreations and generally experience a healthy life filled with happiness and contentment.

Diet: They enjoy pure, clean and fresh food.

Exercise: Their exercise is regulated, and they usually prefer long morning walks or yoga āsanas. They only take up exercises when they understand the benefits.

Activities: They are good at all types of activities. They can pursue anything to perfection and multitask too. But if anything gets out of hand, which is highly unlikely, it can create a lot of health issues.

Rest: They sleep early and get up early without difficulty. Their recreational activities are also regulated. They never waste time on frivolous things.

2. **Kapha Prakṛti** (Kapha is prominent)

Personality: Since kapha represents earth and water elements, people with this nature are generally stout, stable and heavy. The earth element is heavy and provides a lot of stability, like a mountain. People having prominent kapha doṣa are steady in their work, very dutiful and methodical in their approach.

They are not multitaskers, but whatever they do is done with perfection. They are slow to learn, but they grasp well. It takes them time to memorize something, but when they do, they can narrate it down to the last detail. They have calm and peaceful dispositions.

They tend to have large eyes, shiny smooth skin and dense, smooth hair. They are patient and love to persevere. They can sleep easily anywhere. They sleep soundly and tend to snore loudly.

On the other hand, they are prone to laziness and are way too patient. As a result, they often procrastinate and may indulge in self-destructive habits.

Diet: They have a large capacity to eat, though their digestive fire is low. They need to regulate the quantity of food they eat, otherwise they are likely to become obese. They are attracted to food of kapha nature, such as dairy, carbohydrates and sweets. The body takes after its own nature and seeks food made of its own building blocks to maintain and nourish itself. But even slight overeating can lead to imbalanced kapha and weight gain. The activated kapha quickly absorbs food to the body tissues. With weight gain come all the classic problems associated with obesity. First it affects the joints, as the joints are designed to carry a certain load of body weight, then high blood pressure (supplying blood to a larger body requires more pressure and with the heart size remaining the same, the heart experiences a bigger load) leading to cardio complications. But the solution is not to quit all carbs and sweets as their nature needs nourishment from such food. Besides, the mind will remain dissatisfied if such food is not supplied.

So, the only way to maintain the balance is regulation. These regulations include fasting or less eating, combining more of pungent, bitter and astringent tastes (these are foods with a nature opposite to kapha, which are cleaning or flushing agents and discourage one to eat more), reducing sleeping hours, taking up active physical activities and some stressful tasks that force one to work and think. Sāttvic food helps regulate the mind and inspires all of the above said activities to help balance kapha. When kapha is imbalanced, it affects the lungs, throat and sinus. Their food needs to have heating spices, such as ginger and pepper (both are pungent), for aiding digestion and melting down kapha and preventing the ill effects of its excess. Also, the quantity of food can be adjusted by including more hot soups than solids. All these steps are counter to kapha nature and may not be liked by persons with that nature. However, such recommendations help them to counter the excess imbalances. We will come back to this point later in the book.

Exercise: They need to do exercises that make them perspire. They tend to skip their workout because of inertia, though they are the ones who need it the most. Although it's tough for them to perform yoga āsanas, steady practice (which is also natural for them) will help them achieve the unachievable. They are good at sports such as boxing and weight lifting. They are also good at prāṇāyāma (yogic breathing exercises) and meditation—once again, owing to their steady nature.

Activities: They are good at scientific research work, account keeping, artistic (fine art, music and even dance) and creative activities. They also make for good consultants in politics, economics, finance or administration, good teachers and professors, writers or authors, etc. Generally, they don't stress too much as they stay absorbed in their own activities and appear cool and detached in their disposition. They cannot put their heart into something if they don't like it. They may appear very lazy if engaged in such activities. A leader needs to understand what excites them and provide opportunities in those areas.

Rest: Since they do not stress too much, they enjoy good quality rest. But they must adhere to the good advice of not sleeping more than six to seven hours during the night. A daytime nap is also something they look forward to. But it should not be for more than twenty to twenty-five minutes while sitting on a comfortable chair or leaning on a desk, but not lying on a bed.

3. **Pitta Prakṛti** (Pitta is prominent)

Personality: People with this prakṛti/nature will be of medium build. Pitta is represented by the fire and water elements and results in sharp memory and a high intelligence quotient. They are highly analytical, aided by a developed faculty of logic. They work hard, though work is not their first love. Their focus is on the fruit of the labour. They are achievers and don't stop till they achieve the goal. They are highly organized in their work and recreation. They enjoy breaks from work through vacations and other entertainment. They can gain or lose weight just by controlling their diet. Appearance-wise, they tend to have medium-sized, sharp and penetrating eyes and oily skin.

Diet: Their digestive fire is on the higher side. They are attracted to hot and spicy food, including deep-fried savoury dishes. Their taste buds are sharp, and they are very particular about what is being served to them. They become restless when they are hungry. They love protein-rich diets. At a certain point in life, they become conscious about the impact of diet on health and tend to follow diet plans.

Pitta prakṛti people are likely to overeat pitta-stimulating fiery food, thus throwing it out of balance. If they indulge in such food—which has extra fiery chillis and spices—without regulation, they are likely to suffer from chronic gastric disorders. They are also prone to high blood pressure due to their preference for extra salt in their diet.

Their food needs to have pitta-balancing ingredients, spices and herbs. Freshly churned butter, sugarcane juice, coconut water, pointed gourd and neem leaves are coolants. So are spices like turmeric, fennel seeds, clove, mint and cilantro. They should generally reduce the intake of sour and pungent food like raw mango, pepper, asafoetida, chilli, fenugreek seeds, mustard seeds, etc. We will discuss this further in Section Three.

Exercise: People of Pitta prakṛti should ideally exercise till beads of perspiration appear on their forehead. Intense exercise is not recommended for such people, though their tendency is to overdo it. But usually, they are passionate about following routines and that will prevent them from overdoing it. They prefer to go to the gym and shape their muscles instead of doing yoga. If they opt for yoga, it is likely to be power yoga driven by the desire for a flexible and shapely body. They can perform prāṇāyāma (yogic breathing exercises) with practice but struggle with meditation. Some of their favourite sports are lawn tennis, table tennis, badminton and martial arts.

Activities: They are the (aggressive) leaders of the group, no matter the field they are in. CEOs, HODs, admin heads, head teachers or principals often tend to be of pitta-prominent nature. They can work on various projects, but once they decide to take up a task, they prefer to focus on it and lead the team to higher and higher goals. As leaders, they are capable of handling a good deal of stress. But if not regulated, the stress may lead to high blood pressure and end up in strokes that affect the head and the heart. High stress will also adversely affect digestion and sleep. And without proper food and rest, they experience low energy, thus dampening their efficiency, which they hate otherwise.

Sleep: They tend to rest moderately. They never sleep during the day. They may be light sleepers, and their rest is affected by the stress they carry from their work and the food they eat at dinner. But as they are good at maintaining schedules, they can balance diet, rest and exercises with proper guidance.

4. **Vāta Prakṛti** (Vāta is prominent)

Personality: These people are generally skinny, irrespective of their height. They neither gain nor lose weight easily. Because they carry the force of the wind, they are quick to complete tasks. They are very witty. Because of the surplus energy, they are good at multitasking, although prone to committing mistakes. They walk very fast as if they will miss a flight or train and can easily travel a lot. They are very talkative and need to make efforts to check this habit—talking too much also aggravates vāta. They love to move on/change projects, jobs, furniture, mobile phones, houses, interiors of homes, etc. They are quick learners and can learn and speak many languages. They tend to have small, sparkling eyes. Their skin, nails and hair are dry. That's because the vāta or air dries it up. Their body is cool for the same reason. They need regular oil massages with warm oil, preferably mustard oil—which has a heating effect—or sesame oil. Oil should be massaged softly, allowing it to penetrate the skin. Though they are skinny, they enjoy hard massages. However, a hard, vigorous massage will increase the vāta doṣa and thus should be avoided. They are always ready with witty one-liner jokes to entertain their friends. The jokes are also made drily, without too much emotion being expressed; so one needs to be attentive to catch those jokes.

Diet: They like cold and dry food like pani poori (crispy puffed pastries stuffed with mashed potatoes and filled with spicy, sour and sweet water) and bhel (puffed rice mixed with fried/roasted peanuts and corn etc). Though skinny, they can devour a huge quantity of food, and to everyone's surprise, they don't gain any weight. They should top up their food with a good amount of pure ghee (clarified butter) or cold-pressed virgin oil to counter dryness. Sesame oil and olive oil suit this type of prakṛti. Because of their attraction to dry and cold food (like ice cream), they tend to get stomach/abdominal pain, which, if not checked, will lead to various health issues. However, one is attracted to a particular food, driven by one's nature, and it should not be given up completely. The remedy is to regulate the quantity and quality, and back it up with food that has an opposing effect. Thus hot, moist and oily food is good for them and will prevent aggravation of vāta doṣa.

They should avoid bitter and astringent food, which depletes tissues and dries them up. They are prone to constipation due to imbalanced vāta. The air element of vāta also dries the faeces, making it hard and thus difficult to pass. Again, some extra oil helps abate constipation. Some Ayurvedic doctors prescribe castor oil mixed with hot water or hot milk before bedtime in such cases. But if the diet is well-balanced, such medication is not necessary.

Exercise: People of vāta prakṛti are unlikely to gain weight the way those of kapha prakṛti do, but they also do not develop the muscles that pitta prakṛti provides. They are advised to do a minimum amount of exercise as, in general, they are highly active, physically as well as mentally. They are likely to overdo exercises as they carry an extra burst of energy. But too much exercise will take a toll on their already weakened joints and over-exhaust them, causing depletion of tissues. They can effortlessly and quickly learn yoga āsanas. But they struggle with prāṇāyāma and meditation because of a fickle or restless mind. They love cross-country marathons and are also good at long jump, fast bowling in cricket, basketball, etc. They love adventure and sports. To gain weight, they need to focus more on developing muscles rather than accumulating it through fat, and thus may consume more protein to achieve this.

Activities: As mentioned earlier, they are quick learners and can perform multiple tasks. They are spontaneously creative. They excel quickly in any field they apply themselves to. On the negative side, they may end up taking on too many tasks and stressing themselves. They have a strong feeling that they can do anything and may even try doing things that are not their cup of tea, a quality entirely opposite to kapha nature. In other words, they don't mind taking risks. This may create various complications.

Rest: Their mind is restless, and they may miss out on quality rest. They need to relax their mind before going to bed. They can skip daytime naps easily. If rest is not taken care of, it can significantly affect their lifespan. They are prone to high blood pressure, which may affect the performance of their heart and brain. Of all the three prakṛtis we discussed, vāta doṣa-type people need to pay maximum attention to their food and lifestyle (as they inherently tend to neglect it and vāta, carrying kinetic energy, destroys quickly).

5. **Kapha-Pitta Prakṛti** (Kapha and Pitta are both prominent in this prakṛti but it's Kapha-*Pradhān*, i.e., Kapha is more dominating)

They are more likely to follow the rules of kapha without debilitating pitta. This means that they need to find an overlap of kapha and pitta while taking care of themselves. This will be challenging, and as mentioned earlier, when two natures are prominent, they drive us in opposing directions and balancing the doṣas will be tough. In this case while kapha is cooling, pitta is heating, thus making it difficult to balance. But even among the two, one will be stronger than the other. If kapha is pradhān—or the main quality—the digestive force strength may be low and pitta prakṛti will drive us to food that is oily, spicy and loaded with proteins (heavy to digest), thus putting us in difficulty. So, one needs to check and balance the quality and quantity of food accordingly.

6. **Pitta-Kapha Prakṛti** (Pitta and Kapha prominent, but Pitta dominating)

Here, we need to focus more on pitta prakṛti without ignoring the needs of kapha for good health. The problem is similar to the kapha-pitta prakṛti except that pitta is the driving force here. This drive needs to be fine-tuned with the opposing force of kapha.

7. **Pitta-Vāta Prakṛti** (Pitta and Vāta prominent, but pitta dominating)

The pitta makes them love food and the vāta ensures they will have trouble digesting such meals. So, although such pitta-constitution people have a strong craving for fiery fritters, they must control the quantity of such food, especially when vāta is strong—pungent taste aggravates vāta. We will learn more about this in Section Two.

8. **Vāta-Pitta Prakṛti** (Vāta and Pitta prominent, but vāta dominating)

Vāta prakṛti will seek cold food (pani poori), whereas pitta prakṛti may induce a love for hot, steaming food.

9. **Kapha-Vāta Prakṛti** (Kapha and Vāta prominent, but Kapha dominating).

Whereas kapha is stable, vāta is restless. Kapha loves steadiness and vāta loves spontaneity and thus there will be frustration for apparently no reason. For example, while performing a task steadily under the flow of kapha nature, vāta nature may disrupt it by bringing sudden changes or restlessness.

10. **Vāta-Kapha Prakṛti** (Vāta and Kapha prominent, but Vāta dominating)

Here kapha will obstruct the force of vāta.

These are the ten broad classifications of human nature based on the prominence of certain doṣas. But irrespective of which category we belong to, we still are made up of all the three doṣas, and together they shape our life. These doṣas, as a law, always manifest in the order of kapha, pitta and vāta. Every action has three parts: kapha in the beginning, pitta in the middle and vāta in the end. For example, in childhood (*ādi*/beginning), kapha is prominent; in the youth (*madhya*/middle), it is pitta, and in old age (*antya*/end), vāta is prominent. This is irrespective of our tridoṣic nature. With that law come advantages and disadvantages. The advantage of kapha in childhood, for example, is that it builds up the body by combining earth and water elements. The bones, the tissues and muscles, skin and various vital organs—all grow simultaneously and proportionately. All these are aided by the kapha doṣa or prakṛti. But with it comes the problem of nagging cold and cough that usually troubles us during childhood as the more-active kapha tends to be in excess and thus goes out of balance. Similarly, fiery pitta fuels the faculties of intelligence, thoughts and actions of a young man or woman, helping him or her perform and progress. But it can potentially create problems in the digestive canal. Vāta in old age helps the ageing body to maintain the movements of slowing-down limbs and evacuations. But the excess joint pain and restlessness it causes results in inadequate sleep. I remember, in my childhood, my grandpa was always up early in the morning. And then I learnt it's common among ageing people. This is a result of excess vāta.

The conclusion is that any doṣa which is present in excess in one's constitution will cause problems. And it is better to remove them as they accumulate (for example, by including food of an opposite nature). In his book *Prakriti*, Dr Robert Svoboda says that as the three doṣas are so reactive, the body cannot afford to store them for long, any more than a nuclear power plant can afford to keep radioactive wastes on its premises. Kapha is continually expelled from the body via mucus, pitta is regularly excreted through acid and bile and vāta is eliminated both as gas and as muscular or nervous energy. We will see in the future how yogic techniques or kriyās help to remove them from the body and thus bring a balance in the doṣas and good health. Unless doṣas are balanced, we cannot digest properly, even if the food is right according to our nature.

To understand these associated common problems and derive the maximum benefits of a prakṛti—while curtailing all the ill effects—we will need to regulate our diets and daily activities. A growing child's diet will be different from the diet in his/her youth and older age. The sequence of ādi, madhya and antya doesn't end here. This applies universally. For example, during the morning hours, kapha is prominent. So, it should be treated with a light, easy-to-digest breakfast. At noon, pitta takes over and hence the heaviest meal should be around this time. The evening hours signify vāta and are suitable for a moderate amount of fried snacks. The beginning of sleeping hours are characterized by kapha (a cooling and deep sleep), the middle by pitta (disturbed sleep) and the last portion by vāta (sleep quality is poor and various random dreams appear). Finally, this force of vāta kicks one out of bed and simultaneously stimulates the bowels and bladder for evacuation.

Similarly, in sexual intercourse, the beginning part is kapha, the middle is pitta, providing maximum pleasure, and vāta brings forth the climax. The same happens during pregnancy. Vāta in the end helps push the baby out of the womb. The beginning of digestion is dominated by kapha with the slow and regulated release of digestive secretions. The middle is predominated by pitta when actual digestion occurs, and the end of digestion is dominated by vāta when the digested food is pushed through the digestive tract.

This rule applies to the functioning of each cell within our body. Please note, if heavy food is eaten late at night, the pitta phase of sleep will be really disturbed. Cardiac attacks are usually reported during the last phase of sleep when vāta is active. Similarly, asthma attacks occur during the last hours of sleep. These are some general rules we should be aware of. And then, depending upon one's specific doṣa constitution, the diet and activities need to be adjusted to maintain balance and good health. For example, people with vāta constitution should take extra care while going to bed to as their sleep quality is poor compared with kapha constitution.

But the burning question still remains: how do you figure out *your nature*? You must have tried to fit yourself into one of the ten categories using the descriptions of each prakṛti I've provided. You'll also be able to find many questionnaires available online that will help you to determine your tridoṣic nature. One such site is https://www.ayurveda.com/pdf/constitution.pdf. I have also included a short questionnaire later in this section. Once our nature is determined, we can understand our food and work profile better. But before we jump to the questionnaire, we need to understand one more important concept that Ayurveda talks about. This is called *sātmya or* acquired nature.

Sātmya: Acquired Nature

'What gets us into trouble is not what we don't know. It's what we know for sure that just ain't so.'

—*Mark Twain*

When a child is born, he/she should not have anything but mother's milk because the mother fed the child within her womb. Any other food is foreign to the child and may even be fatal. While constantly fighting many negative forces to remain protected from sickness and death, the child gradually shifts to other food, such as grains. Over a period of time, the body starts to accept these 'other foods', and with habitual consumption, the body of the child and the food gradually become one. Food transforms to form our body. Such food, which suits our body because of regular consumption, is called sātmya or accustomed food. Sātmya is a combination of two words *sa* (that) and *ātmya* (very self), which literally means 'non-different from one's own body'. Sātmya food gives comfort to the body. Later, when we want to eat different food, those may cause sickness despite being edible. These are called *asātmya* or 'unfriendly to the self'.

In my hostel in IIT Bombay, where I completed a Masters in Technology, the food would be cooked by a group of Kerali cooks. Somehow, the Kerali food didn't suit my body. Unlike during my childhood, I was no longer the type of person who always fussed about the food that was being served. The cooks were doing their best and the servers were also very friendly, but the food was simply not sātmya to me. Later, while living in Radha Gopinath Ashram in Mumbai, I experienced the same while cooking for monks from different parts of India and the world. Sometimes, the sāttvic food I cooked was not sātmya to them. Visiting monks from far away countries would often fall sick, being deprived of their sātmya food. So, the food habits we develop in our formative years are very important, no matter what our prakṛti or nature is. That food habit becomes our very self and we need to maintain it. But it's best if the child's prakṛti is taken into account (by parents) during the development of the sātmya. Usually, by nature's force, parents do take care of it. But with the availability of so much artificial unseasonal food, one may get confused and overlook this. If sātmya or accustomed food habits are according to our nature, we will be the healthiest.

Sātmya can be even more important than our nature because our body has learnt to accept that type of food and thrives on it too. For example, someone accustomed to eating spicy food, irrespective of their nature, develops the ability to eat it over time. They can eat and digest food even in seasons that it is generally not recommended for. Another example is when an alcoholic person is hospitalized after falling sick and is deprived of alcohol, they may suffer from withdrawal, and medication may not help despite the correct diagnosis. So, doctors administer a regulated dose of alcohol to help the patient recover quickly. Just as grains are not suitable for an infant, alcohol and drugs aren't readily accepted by the body in the beginning.

When I was in university and away from family, once, out of curiosity, I tried to smoke a cigarette. But the experience of the first inhale was so uncomfortable that I decided I would not do it again. I had a similar experience with alcohol. But if one continues to drink and smoke, then those substances become one with our body and it is not advisable to stop having them suddenly.

A long time ago, I watched a documentary where a man plunged his finger into a snake's mouth. The snake bit him, but by the time he took his hand away, the snake clung dead to his finger. His body was more poisonous to the snake. And the snake's poison was sātmya to him. In all these cases, we see people who have made intoxicants (poison) feel welcome in their bodies through habitual consumption.

But as in the case of a baby who is averse to 'other' food in the beginning, yet gradually, with the loving support of the family, adapts to grains and vegetables to the point of sātmya, we can always switch to good habits. So, if we can gradually fall for bad habits, we can gradually also restore good habits.

In our youth, most of us change our habitat by moving to a new geographical location. Our body steadily fights the new sets of opposing forces and creates the necessary sātmya to live peacefully. During my years as a student, I observed certain restaurants on campus would come to life around midnight! After studying long hours in the library or completing an extensive experiment in a lab, students often headed to the restaurants for a break. These places would provide just the right kind of ambience (and wrong food). So, after having noodles and potato chips and gulping down chilled, aerated drinks, the students would return to studies or sleep. I would go to the restaurants too, but it always struck me as odd how someone (including me) could have a proper meal in the middle of the night. In retrospect, I understand that typically, hunger strikes after the mind relaxes from being absorbed in some intense activity that requires your full attention. But hunger in the middle of the night? That sounds pretty odd as we aren't nocturnal creatures. But eventually, the body adapts. So, not only food but also lifestyle can be naturalized as sātmya. Night shifts, burgers and coffee are some other examples. Such habits developed over the years become second nature, or in other words, we develop the necessary sātmya and are at ease with that.

Unfortunately, though we may adapt to a new lifestyle, food or habit, it does not mean it will be good for us. Consistently following something against our nature will lead to trouble at some point. The more we stay closer to our natural state—such as resting at night when it is cooler and working during the day when it is warmer—the healthier we will be. So, if we cannot change our lifestyle for some good reason (such as policemen on night duty), sātmya will help us to cope, but we should try to revert to our nature as much as possible. And when given a chance, we need to gradually return to good habits developed during childhood because those were the years we were closest to our inherent nature.

Now, coming back to knowing your nature. The focus should be on your childhood, especially between the ages of eight and twelve years. Because during this time of our life, we are conscious of our surrounding and its impact on us, yet the brute force to indulge (especially an appetite for sex) has not developed fully. Because when the desire-force is strong, we move under the spell of that passion. Without our knowledge, we move away from regulated nature. On the other hand, these early years can give us a fair sense of our nature or prakṛti. This includes which food you liked, which seasons you found pleasant, which food caused problems, whether you had many friends or just a few but intimate friends, whether you were quick to anger or you forgave easily, which food was enjoyed as well as digested smoothly, which fruit was suitable and which wasn't. Did you sit in the first row of the classroom bench or the second, or middle or last? All these questions will help us understand our nature and guide us to an appropriate food profile and work profile. One needs to be true to oneself while answering the questions (a questionnaire is included below) as that will lead us to our true nature, where we will find our lost comfort.

Doṣa Nirupaṇa Questionnaire (Determining Doṣa-Constitutional Nature)

Before you try to answer the following questionnaire, keep a few things in mind. No doṣa constitution is bad or good. Every doṣa prakṛti has positive as well as negative traits. The idea is to determine your doṣa prakṛti, and strengthen the positive aspects by following the *pathya* or prescribed *āhāra* and *vihāra* (food, activities and recreation) for that particular doṣa constitution. The doṣa prakṛti will push a person equally towards the positive as well as negative aspects of the doṣa constitution which is perfectly natural. But with the strength of this knowledge and applying good intelligence with determination, one should focus and preserve the positive aspect of the doṣa constitution. So, in the questionnaire, when you find questions connected to the negative aspect of a particular doṣa, reflect carefully and answer truthfully. Because the negative traits will also help confirm your doṣa constitution.

Your nature will be the one that you mostly agree with. If two natures are strongly overlapping, the one with more matches will be dominant. If you agree with all three equally, you are the rare person with sama-tridoṣa prakṛti.

1. Body Frame
K (Kapha): I have a broad, heavy and fully-built body.
P (Pitta): I have a medium build with good bulging muscles.
V (Vāta): I am thin and slender with visible veins, joints and thin muscles.

2. Body Weight
K: I gain weight easily and have difficulty losing it.
P: It is easy for me to gain or lose weight (if I decide to do so).
V: I am light and don't gain weight easily.

3. Food
K: I love to eat heavy food full of carbs, protein, fibre and fat.
P: I am attracted to salty and spicy food and have a good thirst.
V: Sometimes I eat a lot, sometimes less.

4. Skin Complexion
K: My skin is thick, moist and smooth.
P: My skin is oily and prone to itching.
V: My skin is dry and skin around feet cracks easily.

5. Hunger
K: My hunger is slow.
P: I feel uncontrolled hunger pangs. When hungry, I must find food.
V: My hunger pattern is erratic.

6. Eating Habits
K: I eat steadily as I relish my food.
P: I eat very fast, thanks to my hunger.
V: I eat very slowly. In a group, I start first and finish last.

7. Walking
K: I walk slowly, one step at a time.
P: I walk at a moderate speed and steadily.
V: I walk very fast.

8. Quality of Hair
K: I have abundant, thick and oily hair.
P: My hair is thin and tends to grey early.
V: My hair is dry, brittle or frizzy.

9. Appearance of Eyes
K: I have large blooming eyes.
P: I have a sharp, penetrating and often intentional gaze.
V: My eyes are small and restless.

10. Flexibility of Joints
K: My joints are large, strong and well lubricated.
P: My joints are loose and flexible.
V: My joints are thin and prominent and have a tendency to pop (with a sound).

11. Soundness of Sleep
K: My sleep is deep and long.
P: I am a moderately sound sleeper, usually needing six hours to feel fresh.
V: I am a light sleeper with a tendency to awaken easily.

12. Body Temperature
K: I am adaptable to most temperatures but do not like cold, wet days.
P: I am usually warm, regardless of the season, and prefer winter.
V: My hands and feet are usually cold and I prefer warm summer.

13. My Temperament
K: I am easy-going, peaceful and supportive.
P: I am purposeful and intense. I like to convince.
V: I am lively and enthusiastic by nature. I like to change.

14. Reaction Under Stress
K: I withdraw and move away.
P: I get angry or aggressive.
V: I become anxious and/or worried.

Tri-Guṇa: Understanding Your Personality

A spider is never captured by its own net. In fact, it is the happiest entity in its net. But the same spider gets badly caught when it enters a cobweb knitted by another spider . . .

The Sanskrit word *guṇa* literally means quality, virtue, excellence or traits. Another meaning of guṇa is rope. *Tri-guṇa* or three qualities of nature, which are all-pervasive, weave (like ropes do) the behavioural traits in us and thus shape our likes and dislikes. These three guṇas, the strings of mother nature, are subtle and classified as *sattva*, meaning goodness, *rajas* referring to passion and *tamas* meaning ignorance. These three modes are the source of pañca mahābhūta (five basic elements) and the tri-doṣas which are made from pañca mahābhūta. Just like numerous stunning paintings can be created using three primary colours, these three guṇas weave a unique masterpiece of personality in each human being. As long as one stays within their nature, one is comfortable, like the spider in its own cobweb. A spider puts a little sticky gum at strategic points in its web, unknown even to other spiders, intending to catch a prey and to safeguard its prey from other spiders. So, we never see two spiders in the same cobweb. Similarly, when one tries to adopt a different nature, unexpected problems will multiply and lead to entanglement. It is crucial to recognize our nature and stay within those boundaries, albeit there is no limit to expanding the boundaries of your particular net.

Not just humans, but all creatures consist of three qualities, in space as well as time. During creation, one of these qualities may manifest more. The entire living world is made up of these bundles of sattva, rajas and tamas. Take for example 'time'. Early morning manifests sattva or goodness. Since we are also made up of sattva, rajas and tamas, time in the early morning hours inspires sattva or goodness in us. This results in a sense of peace and calmness in the early morning hours. We are forgiving, grateful, patient and hopeful for the day. All good qualities naturally manifest in this time frame.

In the same way, daytime is in the mode of passion or raja guṇa. In these hours, we scheme, plan, perform and achieve. To push ourselves to work, we need passion. And the daytime inspires the passion in us to do so. Night hours are *tāmasic*, a time when everything is naturally dark and causes ignorance. And time inspires the tamas in us during the night hours, causing sleep. Sleep causes us to forget ourselves, to the point that whether one is a man or woman. Isn't that a blessing in disguise?

At this point, we can propose two rules:

1. The entire nature is built of sattva, rajas and tamas, including us.
2. When we expose ourselves to a certain quality of nature, then that nature in us gets a boost.

Just as anything else, food can also be *sāttvic, rājasic* or *tāmasic.* Ayurveda recommends always eating sāttvic food. Why so? Ayurveda declares that of these three guṇas, sattva or goodness, as the very term suggests, is the purest (but not perfect). Rajas or passion and tamas or ignorance are impure and cause diseases or bad health. Ayurveda says guṇas are doṣas of the mind and rule it just as tridoṣa rules the body. Triguṇa manipulates subtly and hence is considered more powerful. But you must be wondering, why are rajas and tamas impure?

Let's go back to our example of time in three modes. The night hours are described as tāmasic, because those hours quietly escort us to another unknown world, making us forget about our current existence. Sleep is an essential part of healthy life. So, we are in so much need of tamas or mode of ignorance. It not only rejuvenates the physical body but also relieves our mind. It makes us forget our day's woes and worries. Without a doubt, we need tamas. But then what is impure about tamas? It's easy to fall asleep. All we need is a quiet cool dark place and a bed without bugs. But here is the problem. You may have often found it difficult to get out of a comfortable bed, despite being wide awake. It's as though something is pulling you back to the bed. This inertia and dullness is a negative outcome of tamas or mode of ignorance/darkness. It is a state of negativity. It is so tough, for example, to get kids to go to school in the morning. Occasionally, they pretend to be ill or complain about the school or the teachers. This is all a result of the fact that all kinds of negativities naturally manifest in tamas. So yes, we need tamas, but it potentially brings negativity that can even grow to the extent of denial and depression. This is why Ayurveda classifies tamas as impure. Tamas keeps us away from anxieties for some time, and that helps us rejuvenate our body or health. But that doesn't solve the cause of anxiety. As soon as we are awake, the problem is still there or perhaps has magnified as we didn't do anything about it. Sattva guṇa, on the other hand, helps one to rectify the problems in the awakened stage through the power of knowledge, thus relieving the anxiety once and for ever.

Rajas, or passion, is needed to get us into action mode—getting things done. But once we are into the activity, it is tough to stop. Once we relish the rhythm, it provides an intoxicating kick that is hard to give up. The result is hyperactivity and over-exertion, to the point where we don't even care to sleep! Yes, we forget eating and sleeping, and that's precisely where we start ruining our health. So, the mode of passion is also classified as impure.

Ācārya Vāgabhaṭa, in the very beginning of his classical treatise *Astāṅga Hṛdayam*, has written the following Sanskrit verse:

rāgādi rogān satatānuṣaktān
aśeṣakāya prasrutānaśeṣān
autsukyo moha-aratidāñjadhāna
yo apurvo vaidyāya namostu tasmai

In this verse, the Ācārya pays obeisance to that unique, unparalleled *vaidya* or doctor (referring to Almighty God) who has the ability to uproot the original cause of all the diseases beginning with *rāga*—a strong attachment that arises due to passion and degenerates into lust, greed, pride, anger, envy and illusion (ādi). These negative emotions disrupt the physical functions of our body by causing a lot of anxiety (*autsukya*) and thus affect the overall health, activities and sleep. For example, when we are afflicted with anger, we pant as if we have just finished a 100-metre sprint. Heavy breathing naturally pushes our blood pressure to the higher side and affects our abilities to digest. Who can eat and digest food immediately after a 100-metre dash? The negative emotions comprising lust, greed and pride are impure results of *rajo guṇa* or passion. The other three—anger, envy and illusion (fear), which are more destructive—are the product of tamas or ignorance. In the face of anger, a person forgets who he/she is and does things like hitting someone. That forgetfulness is tamas.

So naturally, triguṇa plays a very vital role when it comes to good health. Yet, there is apparently no dark side of sattva or goodness as it inherently glows with the light of knowledge.* Although we need rajas and tamas for our survival, if we give ourselves over to these lower modes, we will fall sick, and they will eventually reduce our life span.

So, sattva means peace, tranquillity and truthfulness that leads to knowledge, purity and happiness. How does peace lead to knowledge? My spiritual master, His Holiness Radhanath Swami, speaks about one of his personal anecdotes in his autobiography titled *The Journey Home*. In the year 1970, when he was just nineteen years old, through an arduous spiritual, adventurous journey starting from Chicago, he reached the Triveni Sangam in India.

* Except that one may get bound by a sense of contentment arising from the knowledge and resultant happiness that one derives from *sattva guṇa*. Such contentment restricts one's progress in the path of knowledge itself, which would otherwise lead one to *moksha* or liberation.

Triveni Sangam, meaning the confluence of three braids (of rivers), is the point where three holy rivers—Gangā, Jamuna and Saraswati—meet. In his enthusiasm, he decided to swim exactly to the point where the three rivers meet and take holy dips there. So, leaving his belongings on the bank, he jumped into Mother Gangā and swam to the point of confluence. After many fulfilling dips, he started to return. But the swift streams of the Gangā were too strong for him to swim against. Soon he was exhausted and realized he couldn't make it. He looked around desperately for help. In the blazing afternoon sun, there was no one around. But as if it was a godsend, a boatman in a small boat appeared on the horizon. The swami yelled for help. The compassionate boatman came near him. He smiled and thoughtfully stroked his beard. Then he stretched one of his arms at the shoulder level pointing in one direction and left! The struggling swami didn't understand why the man had left him! He kept struggling for a while, only to conclude that death was inevitable. He decided to stop struggling. He thought to himself, 'What better fortune can there be than to die in the holy water of Gangā?' So he let himself go loose and started to submerge in the holy water of Gangā. But within a few moments, it suddenly occurred to him what the boatman (who didn't know English) meant when he signalled with his stretched hand. The boatman was telling him to swim with the flow of the current of Gangā and not against it! In a flash, he started to swim with the current and reached the shore safely. In his struggle and restlessness (mode of passion), he didn't understand that help was extended. But when he was detached and peaceful (mode of goodness), the knowledge was revealed from within. And with the knowledge, he not only could save himself but also experienced gratitude in his heart for the boatman with happiness.

Today's world is extremely interested in work and rest, that is rajas and tamas respectively. But we need sattva or goodness too. Because goodness gives one peace and stability, a platform to analyse good from bad, right from wrong. In other words, sattva helps one to gain the right knowledge that is useful for our existence. Not only that, the balancing ability of sattva can help us regulate our rajas or passion and tamas or ignorance. Regulated passion, such as knowing when to start working and when to stop, is beneficial.

Similarly, regulated ignorance, like regulated sleep, can boost our health. In other words, sattva will preserve the positive side of rajas and tamas. When we expose ourselves to rajas and tamas, our innate rajas and tamas get boosted. Applying the same rule, we can nourish sattva or goodness in us by exposing ourselves to it. For example, if we get up early in the morning, then the natural sattva energy of the morning hours will boost the goodness in us. Sāttvic food will also do the same. A conscious effort to this effect is essential for good health.

At this point, let's remind ourselves that we all need the three guṇas to survive as we are made up of those. Since we ignore or do not nourish sattva in today's world, we place ourselves in danger. Sattva can also bring the best out of rajas and tamas. So we should root ourselves in sattva guṇa.

The next step is to know which triguṇa nature is predominant in you. Just like tridoṣa designs a unique body, triguṇa creates a unique personality. Like each individual has a unique constitutional combination of tridoṣa, each of us is awarded with a unique guṇa. These unique combinations by nature are called *sva-bhāva,* meaning one's own nature. *Bhāva* can be roughly translated as 'tastes' in the sense that each of these guṇa-combinations or qualities inspires some likes or dislikes for certain things or thoughts. Just as there is a broad classification of tridoṣa in which we can place ourselves in a particular category to understand ourselves better, there is a broad classification of triguṇa to understand our personality. This classification helps us to understand our guṇa constitution and we can decide how to bring the best out of it in our work.

This is important to know. Because our activities should be based or driven by our natural qualities. Modern-day education has ignored this to a large extent. A sāttvic person's activities differ from those of rājasic and tāmasic people. Activities based on our nature will keep our mind away from unwanted anxieties, and that in turn keeps our digestive system in order. Activities outside our nature will cause stress which will disrupt the process of digestion. So although the food may be in compliance with our tridoṣa, the body will not be able to process it as the digestive system is not ready. We will discuss more on this in the 'Science of Digestion' section. Below we will discuss in detail people with various categories of nature to help us understand our own.

Classifications of Triguṇa Nature

1. **Sattva (is in prominence)**: People who have sattva in prominence are compassionate, forgiving, truthful, loving, steady in their work and have a flair for cleanliness and austerity (sacrifices for a higher cause). These people are best suited for jobs that cultivate and share knowledge such as teachers, professors, researchers, scientists, judges, advisers to government rulers, priests and even artists of high calibre and thinkers. They are wonderful coaches who inspire. People in this category need not labour hard physically. But they have tough mental resilience and thus can handle a lot of stress. They maintain a spirit of enthusiasm and detachment as they smoothly switch to a lighter mood. Therefore, the diet for such people is usually light and should contain less protein (difficult to digest) and more carbs (easy to digest). The quantity of food should be according to the tridoṣic nature and the force of digestive fire. They are naturally attracted to a sāttvic diet. Usually, people in this category adapt to a simple diet and do not consume many meals. They partake of just enough to keep the body and soul together. On the contrary, their relaxed nature keeps the digestive fire very tidy. They do not need to work out a lot.

A few basic yoga āsanas and prāṇāyāma are good enough for them. But walking long distance in the woods or on mountainous tracks is a pleasant recreation for them. Generally, sattva guṇa connects well with kapha prakṛti and vice versa. Therefore, kapha prakṛti is considered the best among tridoṣa.

2. **Rajas (is in prominence)**: The word rajas has a strong relationship with the word Rājā meaning a king or monarch. In today's world, these are relatable to the positions of CEOs, presidents, ministers, etc. The people with rajas as a prominent quality are rulers/leaders by nature. Raja guṇa refers to passion. Strong passion moves them from within. Yes, kings carry a strong passion to increase land, sovereignty, followers/subjects, etc. They are well built and aggressive. They love to take the credit as the doer or achiever, in giving charity and protecting the innocent. They love to enjoy and are strongly attracted to the opposite sex. A monarch is a natural reveller and has a strong flair for luxury, art, music and the performing arts. They promote all these activities on a large scale as a symbol of development. On the other hand, it is because of these intense luxury-seeking inclinations that they are likely to end up misusing all the wealth and great abilities they are blessed with. Such a desire for enjoyment makes it tough for a person to discriminate right from wrong. Although they have a great capacity to handle stress, when they give in to passionate enjoyment, they lose that capacity. Therefore, for their own benefit and that of the people they lead, they need to heed the advice of sāttvic people. Therefore, a person in power usually consults important personalities before they start the day.

These personalities can be astrologers, Ayurvedic doctors (who guide the cooks) and priests. If they don't place themselves under good advisers, then they will degrade to dictators. A classic example that comes to my mind is that of political adviser Chanakya (375–283 BCE) and Chandragupta Maurya, the unrivalled king of Greater India.

Rājasic people are drawn to rājasic food. Yet they too are advised to adapt to sāttvic food as this food will balance the negative influences of rajas or passion. Sāttvic food will nourish all the positive aspects of a leader. However, the food profile may not be as simple as that of sāttvic people. It has to be according to their build and tridoṣa nature. The food should always be varied, in accordance with their appetite for enjoyment. The food needs to have more protein and the size of the meal should also be large as these types of people are physically very active and have a stronger digestive fire. They can easily ride horses and are heroic in war. They need to do daily heavy exercise or regular gym workouts.

3. **Sattva-Rajas (is in prominence)**: Usually, people with this type of mixed nature are saintly leaders or an ideal CEO. They maintain a spirit of detachment and usually leave a legacy for rulers to follow for many generations. They are attracted to both sāttvic as well as rājasic food, but they prefer and stick to a sāttvic diet as a rule. They eat to perform their duties better, rather than just to enjoy. They voluntarily place themselves under the noble advice of sāttvic sages. They have a disciplined approach to work and recreation and are a rare gift to people they lead. People with high character are naturally attracted to serve with such leaders.

4. **Rajas and Tamas (are in prominence)**: This forms the majority of the population. They mostly belong to the mercantile and working communities. They are driven by the passion that potentially turns to greed and attachment due to the presence of tamas. People in this category do not always know what is best for them. They will be lucky if they find a good leader to work for. They have all the positive as well as the negative qualities associated with rajas and tamas. Again, as with others, they too are advised to stick to a sāttvic diet as it helps in maintaining the positive balance of rajas and tamas in them. If their diet is sāttvic, they will be attracted to wise advice and live happily. Their ability to handle stress is less than that of people in whom sattva is prominent. They need the support of leaders to give their best performance.
5. **Tamas (is in prominence)**: Tamas refers to darkness or ignorance. And in darkness, the immediate experience is fear. When this nature prevails in a person, a sense of insecurity and fear steals their consciousness. They live in doubt. Tamas, more or less, has an impact on everyone's life. At some point, the impact may be severe. But people with tamas in prominence easily fall prey to this influence of fear. Such people always need to perform under the proper care of those with sāttvic qualities or someone with a combination of sattva-rajas. Tamas also means inertia and this quality has a strong attraction for inert objects or materialistic pursuits. People with this type of nature can be some of the finest artists, musicians, engineers, architects, scientists and doctors. You will find people with sattva guṇa and rajo guṇa also in these professions, but the difference is in the ability to digest the amount of

stress. Sometimes an artist in tamas can perform better than an artist in the mode of goodness (sāttvic artist) if protected against fear by a good teacher/coach or a leader. When leaders try to exploit such people, their insecurity merely increases and their delicate faith is shattered. The result is either they withdraw or revolt. Withdrawal may lead them to destructive addictions like alcohol, drugs, pornography, etc. If not properly guided, then the tamas quality can degrade one to destroy. However, what is really positive about people in tamas is the strong faith they carry for the people who care for them. When in genuine care, they can happily give their very life away for such leaders. So, people in tamas need to be careful while choosing a leader to work with. A sāttvic or rājasic selfless leader can bring the best out of them. A tāmasic leader can lead them down the path of destruction. Tāmasic people too are recommended sāttvic diet, because tāmasic diet by nature is destructive. So, if they fall for tāmasic diet, which is likely to attract them, it will simply increase the level of their insecurity and fear. As a result, they may fall into depression, compromise on their life's quality and eventually shorten their life span. A sāttvic diet, on the other hand, can help them keep sattva alive and which in turn helps them, for example, to find a good sāttvic leader to work with.

6. **Sattva and Tamas:** This combination is unlikely to happen. It's like trying to find a shadow in bright light or vice-versa.

You can have a fair amount of understanding about your nature based on the above description about triguṇa. Now combine this with the result of the Doṣa Nirupaṇa questionnaire to understand one's guṇa and doṣa prakṛti or nature.

Conclusion

We started this section with the objective of understanding and preparing a personalized food profile. We discussed how to understand our own psycho-physical nature using Ayurvedic concepts of tridoṣa and triguṇa. Once we know our nature, we will map this nature to the tridoṣa and triguṇa nature of the food we need to consume. This leaves us to understand the triguṇa and tridoṣa nature of food. The following sections will guide us on what food an individual should eat and what one shouldn't. In other words, we will create a food profile based on our guṇa and doṣa. We will try to emphasize more on the principles and understand them with a few examples. Once we know the principles, we can fairly apply those to any cuisine and for any time, climate and country.

Before we conclude this section, we must emphasize that no nature, based on guṇa and doṣa, is inferior or superior. Every nature has a certain function in relation to the cosmos we live in and when we look at the bigger picture, we appreciate this more and more. Even a tiny screw in a large machine has a critical role in holding the tools together and helps the machine work smoothly. Every nature operates best under certain situations. When everyone performs their tasks sincerely, each one of them naturally attracts the appreciation and affection of others. This keeps one above pettiness and creates a sublime atmosphere of inner peace, happiness and satisfaction.

Section Two

Rasa Science

Ṣaḍrasa: Six Tastes
Guṇas: Qualities of Food Ingredients
Vīrya: Potency of Food Ingredients
Vipāka: After-Effects of Digestion

Rasa Science

'Go for vitality, not comfort.'

—Nicholas Lore

I remember visiting my mother's remote village as a child. It had no electricity then. It was surrounded by beautiful lakes and green vegetation for miles in all directions. The vegetables from those farms were full of *rasa,* or juices. The moment we cut the vegetables, the juices oozed out. This was a mark that those vegetables were full of life. Such fresh foods were bountifully surcharged with *prāṇa-śakti*, or vitality. Each day's meals would be planned around whichever fresh vegetables the farmers would bring in their beautifully woven bamboo baskets. Life was simple. Sometimes, seasonal supplies would have little variety of vegetables, yet thanks to the rich traditional cooking, it didn't seem monotonous. Using one simple ingredient, one could cook it in many different ways, by combining different spices and tastes, and at the same time, make it doṣa-friendly. Such cooking techniques would not only impart a rich taste, but also a lot of goodness that was beneficial for the body as well as the mind.

Ironically, today it is tough for people living in a metropolis to decide what to eat on a given day as they are surrounded by numerous options. Usually, people end up cooking what they enjoy the most. The variety and freshness of seasonal food are often skipped.

To add to it, in the age of convenience, everyone seems to be a bit callous about how they cook their food. Instead of cooking fresh food for a meal, we tend to cook in advance and stock it up in the fridge. In fact, cooking is often a low priority for most people, and there seems to be no time to cook at home. Hence, food stores are filled with frozen pre-cooked food.

Scientists first invented pre-cooked, preserved food for brave soldiers guarding the borders, those travelling in submarines or spaceships (astronauts), and people conducting research on the icy poles. Such food is meant to sustain life under challenging circumstances. But for a person with easy access to fresh food, it is not a good option and can only be harmful in the long run.

The alternative to consuming pre-cooked, packaged and frozen food is to rethink the role your kitchen plays in your life. Nothing can be learnt without training, including cooking. When we cook some entrées successfully, an air of excitement certainly fills the kitchen and our lives. Food is ingested by our bodies. Just think how careful we need to be to plan and execute a menu. So never mind cleaning up the dishes. Or hire someone to clean up the kitchen, in case you are too busy. It's better to pay for someone's living than to spend on fighting sickness.

One of my friends living in the Bay Area of Silicon Valley in California, USA, decided to remove all pre-packaged and pre-cooked food from their home and instead eat fresh, home-cooked food every day. Their kitchen turned from a quiet spot into a space that brought the family together. Earlier, it would be a daily struggle to get the kids (aged five and ten) to finish their meals. But when the parents began cooking, the kids took an interest and were excited to try out the new dishes. What surprised the adults was that the kids enjoyed the food better, and they had to put no extra effort into getting them to eat. In fact, the kids started looking forward to mealtimes.

Preparing nutritious food is not just about picking the right ingredients but also about cooking them the right way so the food can be digested well by the body. Unless one is guided by the tradition or wisdom of Ayurveda, our own faulty cooking can take us down the path of ill health. One of the most important things in this regard is to know the nature of seasonal ingredients and their properties. The other, which we will discuss later, is the process of cooking itself.

Qualities of Food Ingredients

Each ingredient has many properties that one should be aware of before deciding to cook with it. In Section Three, we will discuss the tridoṣa and triguṇa nature of food. Yet, we need to know a few more qualities of food ingredients before we get there as the tridoṣa nature of food ingredients is affected by these qualities. Here we will discuss those qualities/properties. Armed with this knowledge and then the tridoṣa nature of food ingredients, we will have a complete understanding of how food can be cooked and digested properly. These essential properties of food ingredients that one needs to be aware of are:

1. Ṣaḍrasa or Six Tastes: Sweet or Sour, etc.
1. Guṇa or Qualities: Heavy or Light, Dry or Oily, etc.
2. Vīrya or Potency: Hot or Cold
3. Vipāka (Taste After Digestion): Sweet, Sour, etc.

Ṣaḍrasa: Six Tastes

Taste is more than just a sensation. Caraka-Saṃhitā says a physician who has good knowledge of tridoṣa and ṣaḍrasa or six tastes can treat any disease effectively. The quality of an ingredient can be identified just by its taste. For example, if an ingredient is pungent (fiery hot), it will generally increase or activate pitta doṣa, be easy to digest and cause dryness, etc. In this way, from taste itself, we can understand the impact on digestion, tridoṣa and health.

Rasa is an experience or something that inspires a particular mood, thus contributing to our feelings and manifests various sentiments, such as happiness, anger and frustration. When rasa flows into us, it quickly influences us by expanding into our body, senses, mind and heart. In the Bhagavad Gitā, Krishna says, 'Of all the rasas, I am water.' Water is neither sweet nor salty or sour. Water is just water, yet it carries a taste, and that is rasa. No drink can quench our thirst like water. Pure, clean water is not only nourishing to the body but also touches and purifies our mind. Many Ayurvedic preceptors believe that all the rasas originate in water, as much as all colours are present in white colour. Rasa is roughly translated as taste in English, although it means much more. The word that corresponds to taste in Sanskrit is *svādu* and only partially represents rasa. Rasa is more sublime in its influence than taste. Without rasas, you would not be able to determine the essence of food.

What are the Six Rasas? The six tastes are sweet, sour, salty, pungent, bitter and astringent. These tastes are detected by the taste buds on the tongue and transported by the water content in each ingredient. Different types of taste buds are spread throughout the tongue: the tip hosts both the sweet and salty taste buds, the sides of the front portion host the sour ones, the sides of the rear portion host the pungent ones, and the centre rear part (closer to the throat) hosts the astringent taste buds. The arrangements are illustrated in Figure 2.1 below.

Figure 2.1

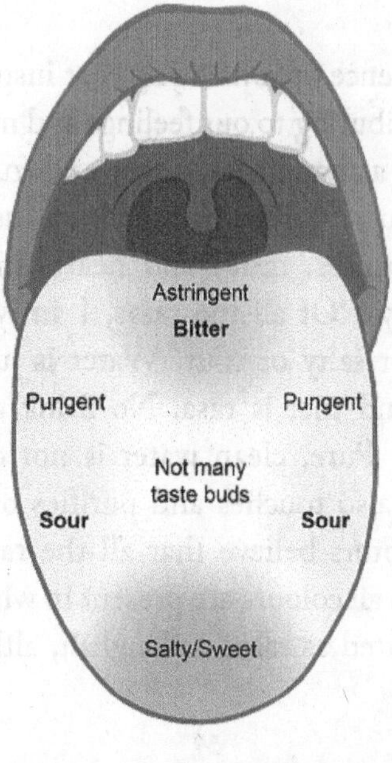

Food with sweet or *madhura* taste is always welcome and forms the major portion of our diet. When I say sweet taste, it refers to all food with natural sugar, and need not be predominantly sweet to taste. For example, rice, corn and wheat have a natural mild sweetness. So do vegetables, such as pumpkin and potatoes. If we look at a typical meal, we will find these food ingredients form the predominant portion of the meal. As the nutrients from such food are essential to build tissues, sweet taste buds are at the front tip of the tongue to help easily detect such food.

Salt regulates the water content of the body and needs to be consumed in lesser quantities than food with a sweet taste. Salt is added to sweet-tasting food like fried potato chips. Too much salt leads to too much water in the body as salt attracts water through osmosis. Excess water causes obesity and blood pressure to rise. However, sodium from salt plays an important role in muscle contraction and nervous movement. An average adult needs around 6 gm of salt a day. So, we cannot remove it altogether from our diet. While discussing the tridoṣa nature of food ingredients, we will talk about various other benefits of different types of salt.

Foods with a sour taste, which mostly aid in digestion, need to be consumed in smaller doses than those with sweet taste. Even a slight increase in salty and sour taste can be unhealthy. Lemon juice, tamarind, raw mangoes, pomegranate, kokam and Indian gooseberries are some examples.

Pungent ingredients should be consumed in moderation. A few examples of pungent ingredients are chilli peppers, black pepper and ginger.

These four tastes are loved universally. Although pungency may not be welcomed by all, many people love it.

Some of the Thai, Indian and Mexican cuisines are loaded with chilli peppers.

Foods with bitter and astringent taste are not so welcome. But they act as essential cleansing agents. Cleansing agents are required in small doses, and the buds that recognize these tastes are situated at the back of the tongue (near the throat). By the time one can register these tastes, which may be a bit unpleasant to some, it is too late to reject it, and we gulp it down like medicine. Medicines are essential but cannot be part of our main diet. The buds for the sour and salty taste, which is less prevalent in our diet than sweet taste, but more than bitter or astringent, are on the sides of our tongue. All these taste buds get activated when all tastes are present in our diet and thus promote digestion to the fullest. Therefore, Ayurveda recommends that all the tastes should be part of our meal. The ingredients with a sweet taste should form the biggest portion, followed by salty, sour, pungent, bitter and astringent. The order of eating should also follow from sweet to astringent taste. Because sweet taste comprises earth and water elements, it is heavy to digest and thus should be consumed in the beginning when hunger is the most extreme. Sweet taste generally comes with salty and sour taste and forms the first part of our meals. Pungent, bitter and astringent are easier to digest and should be eaten towards the later part of the meal.

Production of Rasa/Tastes: The various rasas/tastes in different ingredients result from different interactions between the five great elements. In Section One, we understood how these elements combine to form tridoṣa. Similarly, they combine to form six tastes.

It is natural then that all six tastes also affect the doṣas because of these common elements. This is shown in Table 2.1.

Table 2.1: Origin of Taste and their Effect on Doṣas

Taste/Tridoṣa	Origin	Effect on Doṣas
Sweet/Kapha	Earth + Water	Kapha↑; Pitta and Vāta ↓
Sour	Earth + Fire	Kapha and Pitta↑; Vāta ↓
Salty/Pitta	Fire + Water	Kapha and Pitta↑; Vāta ↓
Pungent	Fire + Air	Vāta and Pitta ↑; Kapha ↓
Bitter/Vāta	Air + Space	Vāta↑; Kapha and Pitta↓
Astringent	Space + Earth	Vāta↑; Kapha and Pitta↓

Effect of Rasas on Our Tridoṣa: Generally, the first three rasas—sweet, sour and salty—increase kapha due to the earth and water elements, and balance or reduce vāta doṣa due to a lack of the air element. The opposite is done by the remaining three rasas—pungent, bitter and astringent—as they have space and air elements, opposite to the nature of the earth element (air has no shape, earth has a definite form). Although astringent has the earth element, it pacifies or reduces kapha due to the dryness caused by the space element. Pungent, salty and sour rasas containing the fire element increase pitta doṣa (which intrinsically has the fire element) and sweet, bitter and astringent rasas, lacking the fire element, balance pitta doṣa. This is shown in Table 2.1 and Chart 2.1. This is important to know and helps us understand what can be eaten and what is to be avoided for certain doṣa constitutions and when we experience an imbalance in certain doṣas. Let's look at this more closely.

Chart 2.1: Effect of Tastes on Doṣas

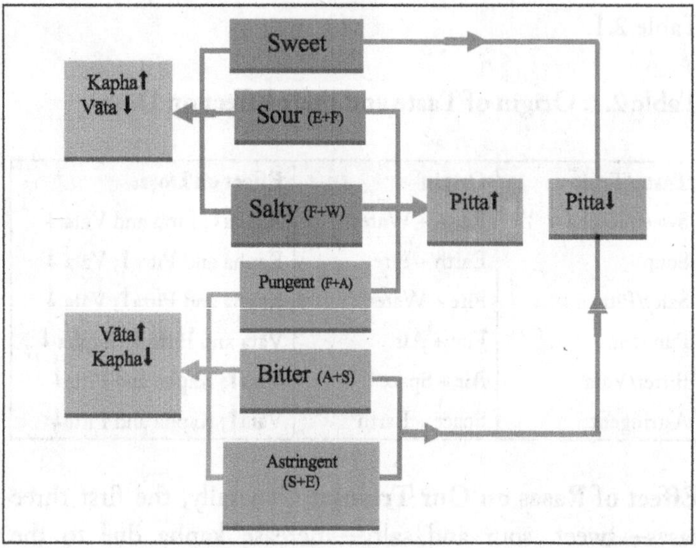

Characteristics and Impact of Rasas

Sweet Taste (Madhura) K↑P↓V↓: As mentioned above, when we discuss sweet taste, it refers to all ingredients that naturally have a small amount of sugar. These may not necessarily be confectionery items. It usually refers to food such as rice, corn, potatoes and pumpkin. This type of food and preparation is typically characterized as follows:

As sweet taste is attractive to the palate, one tends to have a mouthful of it. It provides a feeling of contentment and pleasure to the body and senses.

Impact on the Body and Tridoṣa: Food with this taste is nourishing. Sweet rasa lends strength to the tissues and is very important for growing kids, the aged and the wounded. It is also valuable for the vitality of hair and sense organs and enhances *ojas* (aura or effulgence). It increases breast milk and helps heal broken limbs. Such food supplies the energy for all our activities and prolongs life.

Because of the inherent unctuousness, the sweet taste balances vāta doṣa. Because of the lack of fire element, it also balances pitta. However, such food is generally heavy due to the overarching presence of the earth element and thus is difficult to digest. People with poor digestive fire will not be able to fully assimilate the nourishment provided by food with this taste. And when madhura rasa is not digested or is present in excess in the body, it leads to various health problems related to fat and kapha doṣa. As a result, one may be at risk of obesity, diabetes, enlargement of glands in the neck, etc. People of kapha prakṛti, who are naturally attracted to this type of food, must regulate the quantity and exercise daily.

Impact on the Mind: This taste imparts a sense of satisfaction to our mind. Thus, it is considered sāttvic and is rooted in kapha prakṛti. In some traditions, sweets (desserts) are offered towards the end of the meal so that the mind's craving ceases and a person feels satisfied. However, since food with a sweet taste is heavy to digest and dessert is eaten at the end of a meal, it should be consumed in small quantities. On the other hand, if one eats sweets in the beginning, one will feel satiated early and not be able to relish other food and tastes. Madhura rasa also instils gratitude and thus nourishes and strengthens our memory. It is said that cow milk, which has madhura taste in prominence, nourishes the fine tissues in the brain to enhance memory.

Sour Taste (*Amḷa*) K↑P↑V↓: This taste makes the mouth salivate excessively. Even the thought of a sour pickle makes the mouth water. It causes a tingling sensation in the teeth as well and makes you shut your eyes tightly.

Impact on the Body and Tridoṣa: Amḷa means acid. All sour food is more acidic in nature, a result of the fire element in it. Thus, sour taste—which stimulates the digestive power or pitta doṣa—is a good appetizer, which ignites the digestive system and hunger. Sour food is hot in potency* (creates heat in the body after being consumed) though it may be cold to the touch (for example, pickle). It relieves burning sensation upon external application (for example, tamarind), satiates the senses and causes salivation while chewing such food, which aids in digestion. Food with sour taste moves the choked vāta downwards, which is good for evacuation. This type of food should be regulated carefully, as it can cause the pitta doṣa to spike, resulting in various health problems, such as hyperacidity.

Being on predominantly sour food can make the muscles flabby or loose, leading to loss of strength, itching, blindness, excessive thirst and fever. All these happen due to excessive pitta imbalance. Therefore, we must regulate the quantity of sour taste in our food.

Sour taste, which results from the fire element, is all-pervasive (delocalized) in our body in the form of heat, and balances excess kapha. Kapha, on the other hand, is an example of localized energy stored in tissues. Pitta is a readily

* Potency is the functional capacity of a substance. When we say that potency is hot, it means the food eaten will create heat in the body. We will discuss more about potency later in this section.

available pure active energy and our body utilizes it to process all the incoming inputs, which includes not just food but also information such as sight, touch, sound and thoughts. When our body processes any or all of these inputs, pitta 'digests' and assimilates the essence to nourish and build us (and waste is also created as a by-product). So, when pitta goes out of balance, even our mind and intelligence will not function at the optimum level.

Since pitta is significantly involved in the digestion process, it can affect the entire body when out of balance. Moreover, as it is delocalized and connected throughout, it'll impact multiple aspects, and the result could even be bitter feelings, anger and frustration. Thus, one should consume food with a sour taste in considerably lesser amounts than food that is sweet and regulate the intake very carefully.

It is also worth mentioning here that even if the food you eat is not pure or decomposed, pitta will still try to digest it, which can cause health problems. Similarly, if other inputs such as touch, sight, sound and thoughts are not pure, then pitta will process them and nourish the negativities in us. For example, if we are surrounded by critical and negative people and pay attention to them, we tend to become critical and fault-finding.

Impact on the Mind: Sour taste stimulates intellectual activities, especially in relation to logic and analysis. People of pitta prakṛti are good at analysis, be it business or software programming. But a diet loaded with sour taste will activate the pitta and thus make the analytical trait stand out. The south Indian diet, which is generally flavoured with tamarind and other souring ingredients, activates pitta. It may even be a reason that many people from the south Indian states tend to have an interest in studying software and analytics.

Salty Taste (*Lavaṇa*) K↑P↑V↓: Salty taste causes excess salivation in the mouth and can lead to a burning sensation on the cheeks and throat.

Impact on the Body and Tridoṣa: Salt removes rigidity and activates the nervous system. Salt clears blockages in pores or channels as liquids flow from low to high concentration of salt (osmosis). Salt increases digestive activity, improves the taste of food, causes sweating, penetrates deep into the tissues, causes bursting of the abscesses (boils) and lubricates (because it attracts moisture).

Excess salt increases pitta and vāta doṣas and causes imbalance. The increased pitta promotes piles and bleeding in the nose. Imbalanced vāta creates wind in the digestive tract (this may result in disrupted digestive fire, constipation, etc.). Other effects of excess salt are baldness, greying of hair, wrinkled skin, thirst and diminishing strength.

Impact on the Mind: Salt creates a sense of craving. For example, it is difficult to stop snacking on potato chips. We don't stop eating till only crumbs remain, for which we search the corners of the packet. Still, a sense of dissatisfaction continues. Salt instils greed in the mind and can cause one to overeat.

Pungent (*Katu*) K↓P↑V↑: Pungent taste (hot chilli for example) stimulates or excites the tongue. It causes irritation in and secretions from the eyes, nose and mouth. It also causes a burning sensation.

Impact on the Body and Tridoṣa: Pungent taste keeps the mouth and throat clean (traditional classical singers chew black pepper with sugar candy to keep the throat clean and healthy), promotes digestion and easy absorption of food, and helps in eliminating food after digestion (due to downward movement of the increased vāta). People who eat spicy food, as in most parts of India, tend to suffer less from constipation, as the food is well spiced with chilli peppers, black pepper or ginger. Because of its ability to dissolve kapha doṣa, food with pungent taste clears blood clotting and other similar obstructions (so, it is good for the heart). Also, the fiery nature melts the accumulated or aggravated kapha (which can present as cough and cold).

Excessive consumption of pungent taste in food destroys virility, causes emaciation, asthma and burning sensation in the throat, produces excessive heat and thirst and diminishes bodily strength. It also causes pain in the waist and back.

Impact on the Mind: Pungent taste opens up all the channels in the body, including the mind. It treats the stubbornness of the mind and allows one to look at other alternatives. This is also an intellectual stimulus. When I was a kid, I was not so good at maths. One of my uncles suggested I ate chilli peppers. So, I started increasing my chilli consumption when I was in 7th/8th grade. My skill at maths gradually improved and I stood second in maths in my Std Ten board exams!

Bitter Taste (*Tikta*) V↑K↓P↓: Bitter taste is responsible for cleansing the mouth and overpowering the taste buds, which block out other tastes.

Impact on the Body and Tridoṣa: Inherently bitter food is an excellent antiseptic and cures worm (bacteria, parasites, etc.) infestations. Because it is an effective pitta-balancing rasa, it cures many diseases caused by imbalanced pitta, such as burning sensation, skin irritation, fever, nausea, throat irritation, etc. Some of these diseases might be due to kapha imbalance (like fever and throat infection), which is also balanced by a bitter taste. It cleanses the digestive canal effectively and re-establishes the digestive fire. Because it is kapha balancing, it is very effective in removing fat and obesity. It also purifies breast milk, dries up moisture and increases intelligence.

When bitter food is consumed in excess, vāta will go out of balance, thus causing excessive loss of tissues, depleted plasma, muscle, fat, bone marrow and semen. So, bitter food should be eaten in tiny portions or infrequently, less than food with sour and salty rasas. Otherwise, loss of *dhātus*/tissues will lead to loss of strength, emaciation, impotence or loss of sexual vigour, etc.

Impact on the Mind: Bitter food quells cravings and can be effective for people who have a tendency to overeat or give in to temptation.

Astringent Taste (*Kaṣāya*) V↑K↓P↓: This inactivates the entire tongue, completely diminishes all other tastes and causes obstructions in the throat passage. Although this taste is similar in nature to bitter taste in terms of its impact on tridoṣa, the difference is that food with kaṣāya or astringent taste is difficult to digest.

Impact on the Body and Tridoṣa: Astringent taste is similar to that of a raw plantain peel. Food with this taste generally mitigates pitta and kapha and is an excellent cleansing agent. It cleanses the blood and helps heal wounds by naturally drying moisture. It obstructs digestion and absorbs water from the waste, which can cause constipation. This obstruction, however, is important as it prevents excess secretion of digestive juices. Usually, acidity or heartburn occurs due to excessive secretion from digestive glands. So *tāmbula* or paan (betel leaf) is generally offered at the end of a typical Ayurvedic meal. Tāmbula is a pack of paan leaf with a thin coat of lime paste (calcium bicarbonate), some spices like clove, and betel nut as main ingredients. The lime helps balance the excess acidity (post-digestion pitta) in the stomach, thus preventing heartburn. The astringent taste in betel nuts prevents or seals further secretion of digestive juices. Unfortunately, adding dry chewable tobacco ruins the paan. Tobacco is not only addictive, it is also known to cause diseases, such as mouth cancer. Remember that paan is supposed to be eaten at the end of the meal. Of course, it will have a harmful impact if it is eaten addictively throughout the day.

Wikipedia categorizes betel nut as carcinogenic. But it has been used in moderation for hundreds of years in India without side effects. Astringent food is not for indulgence. Excessive consumption causes severe indigestion, flatulence, pain in the heart region due to increased vāta doṣa and resultant increase in wind (*vāyu*), unquenchable thirst, loss of virility, emaciation and constipation. However, with a proper understanding, this tradition of incorporating astringent taste beneficially can again be brought back into practice. In eastern Indian tradition, when a marriage is fixed, families exchange betel nuts and paan leaf to indicate the cementing of the relationship.

Impact on the Mind: Astringent taste banishes the lethargy of the mind as it pushes the vāta prakṛti. So, if you often feel like napping after a meal, this can help prevent that. As astringent taste also curbs the desire to eat, it prevents overeating. No one craves a samosa or a slice of pizza after having paan.

Conclusion

Of all the qualities of food, rasa or taste is the basis. No other quality will be as defining a characteristic as taste. By knowing rasa, one can decide when to eat what, the sequence of eating and how much to eat to balance a particular imbalanced doṣa. Also, knowledge of rasa science helps to take care of certain doṣa constitution. For example, pitta prakṛti people should consume less of sour taste and more of sweet taste. Similarly, vāta-prakṛti persons or those with excess imbalanced vāta should avoid excessive bitter taste.

But we should also be aware of the exceptional qualities of some ingredients, which take precedence above the general rules. For example, food ingredients of madhura rasa or sweet taste are heavy to digest, but not aged sali rice, green moong and honey. Sour taste increases pitta, but pomegranate, lemon or gooseberries don't have that effect. It is confirmed by modern medical findings that although gooseberries are sour and acidic in their raw state, post digestion, they become alkaline. Table 2.2 lists some of those examples as given by Vāgabhaṭa in his classic Ayurvedic treatise *Astāṅga Hṛdayam*, which has been considered an authoritative book by Ayurvedic doctors for many centuries.

Table 2.2: Examples of Six Tastes with Exceptions

Taste/Rasa	Examples	General Properties	Exceptions
Sweet/ Madhura	Ghee, jaggery, grapes, rice, wheat, gold metal, corn, etc.	Heavy to digest, kapha increasing	Aged sali rice, green moong beans and godhūma wheat, honey and rock-candy sugar (misri)
Sour	Tamarind, gooseberry, pomegranate, yoghurt, butter milk, silver metal, raw mango, etc.	Increases pitta, hot in potency	Pomegranate, gooseberry
Salty	Saindhava (rock salt), black salt, sea salt, lead metal, etc.	Bad for eyes	Saindhava
Bitter	Bitter gourd, neem, potala (pointed gourd), kansa metal, iron metal, sandalwood	Non-aphrodisiac	Pointed gourd
Pungent	Asafoetida, chilli pepper, black pepper, ginger, etc.	Non-aphrodisiac	Dried ginger (sunthi)
Astringent	Raw plantain, honey, dates, coral and pearl pots, etc.	Cold and obstructive	Abhayā

Guṇas: Qualities of Food Ingredients

These guṇas we speak of here are not the triguṇa we have discussed. Sometimes triguṇa is described as mahāguṇa or the greater universal guṇa from which all other guṇas or qualities manifest. Ayurveda speaks of specific attributes of food ingredients (and medicines) that can help fine-tune our food profile. These qualities help us to understand the peculiarities of the food ingredients we use. You may ask, 'Why are doṣa and rasa insufficient in describing food ingredients? How much more do I need to know?' So far, we have discussed doṣa and rasa in their pure forms. But in reality, each food ingredient is produced by a unique combination of earth, water, air, fire and ether. On the other hand, the food ingredient has its own specific identity and qualities. These are intrinsic to that ingredient and cannot be separated from it. The beauty is that the unique combinations can produce two or more tastes in one ingredient. For example, moong is both sweet and astringent. Now different rasas/tastes will affect doṣas differently and thus can either create a positive situation (symphony) or negative (cacophony/diseases). However, each ingredient has some overarching qualities. Each of those qualities has a specific action that affects our digestion, doṣas and ultimately, health. So one needs to understand the qualities of each ingredient. These can be understood by direct repeated observations (*pratyakhṣa pramāṇa* or direct evidence).

The quality of an ingredient is determined by the presence of one strong element and is evaluated by perception (smell, taste, form, touch and sound). So say, a group of ingredients that has earth as the major element will have earthly qualities. So in this way, Ācārya Vāgabhaṭa has grouped five categories of ingredients based on the five basic elements (pañca mahābhūta) and described their characteristics (Table 2.3). Vāgabhaṭa says ingredients having fiery and airy nature will move upward and those of earthly and watery nature will move downward.

Table 2.3: Five Major Categories of Qualities

Guṇa/ Quality	Major Element	Characteristics/ perceptibility	Bestows	Example
Earthly	Earth	Heavy, bulky, stable, perceptible by smell	Compactness, heaviness and growth	Rice, sweets
Watery	Water	Heavy, flowy, cold, unctuous/ oily, dull, dense and perceptible nature is watery	Lubrication, secretion, keeping wet, satiation and cohesion	Milk
Fiery	Fire	Dry, penetrating, hot, non-slimy, subtle, noticeable feature is fiery form	Burning sensation, lustre, expression of colour, digestion (transformation and putrefaction)	Chilli pepper

Guṇa/ Quality	Major Element	Characteristics/ perceptibility	Bestows	Example
Airy	Air	Dry, non-slimy, light, perceptible by touch sensation	Dryness, lightness, transparency, movement/ activity and exhaustion	Puffed rice
Spatial	Sky	Minute, transparent, light and perceptible by sound	Cavitation/ hollowness, lightness/ weightlessness	Herbal smokes

Vīrya: Potency of Food Ingredients

The word *vīrya* (potency) derives from the word vīra—a person with valour who naturally loves action. That which is responsible for action of an ingredient is called vīrya.

Fresh food is more potent than stale food. Potency is the active energy that acts for a certain period. Loss of freshness is proportional to loss of action on our doṣas. For example, it is observed that a drug/medicine that works effectively on doṣas and tissues becomes ineffective if left aside for some days. The drug's composition may remain the same. Or in other words, it loses the potency to act, just as a warrior loses the potency to fight after a while. So, Ayurveda strongly advises that we eat fresh food to benefit from the potency. Thus, it is best to cook vegetables when they are fresh and eat grains that haven't been cooked for long. Potency acts irrespective of guṇa (qualities) or rasa (tastes) and sometimes overrides them. So, it is important to look for potency, also called the prāṇa-śakti or vitality of the food.

Vāgabhaṭa focuses on the eight qualities that fall under the category of vīrya or potent, and we should focus on these in our day-to-day diet. When qualities become responsible for the action or the functional capacity of an ingredient, then it falls under the category of vīrya or potency. These are heavy, light, hot, cool, oily, dry, soft (malleable) and penetrating. We have discussed these eight potent qualities in Table 2.4. But of all these qualities, two are considered by many authorities as the ones contributing most to the potencies. These are hot and cool. Because these two qualities are based on agni (fire or sun) and *soma* (cooling moon planet), they are the major movers or relaxers in our life. Fire spends energy and makes things move. On the other hand, a cooling rest allows gaining of strength. So, both awakening and sleeping result from the potency of the sun and moon and are important in our lives. All other potencies fall between awakening and sleeping, and are thus considered subsidiary potencies. So, if we classify the potency of ingredients in terms of hot or cool, it would help us to understand our requirement precisely. Naturally, food with hot potency should be avoided during dinner. But remember, for the potency to be effective, the food needs to be fresh and sāttvic.

Table 2.4: Examples of Typical Guṇa or Qualities

Quality	Impact on Doṣa	Related Rasa/ Taste	Impact on Digestion
Heavy	Increases kapha	Sweet, salty	More time to digest
Light	Decreases kapha	Sour	Easy to digest
Cool	Increases vāta	Sweet, bitter, astringent	Bitter is easy to digest
Hot	Increases pitta	Sour, pungent, salty	Easy to digest
Oily	Decreases vāta	Sweet	More time to digest
Dry	Increases vāta	Astringent	Difficult to digest
Soft	Increases kapha	Sweet, salty	More time to digest

Quality	Impact on Doṣa	Related Rasa/ Taste	Impact on Digestion
Penetrating	Increases pitta	Pungent	Easy to digest

Hot and Cool Vīrya:

Hot potency (*usṇa* vīrya) produces giddiness, thirst, perspiration and exhaustion (without any work, for example after biting a hot fresh green chilli pepper) and burning sensation. So such food should be handled carefully and as per the need. Food with hot potency gets cooked quickly (transformation) and mitigates vāta and kapha.

Cool potency helps in production of tissues, gives life (the kind we get after a solid rest), and ability to withhold or stop (for example from reacting angrily). It also purifies blood and pitta.

Conclusion

Thus we have listed eight prominent guṇas or qualities. These are whether the ingredient is heavy or light to digest, whether it creates heat in the body or cools it down, whether it is dry or oily and whether it is soft or penetrating. Like taste, all these eight qualities also affect our doṣa balance and digestion. For example, cheese belongs to kapha prakṛti and requires strong digestive fire and time to digest. Moong dal is light to digest. Chilli pepper is hot, whereas mint is cooling. Puffed rice is dry, whereas milk is unctuous or oily. Salt is penetrating and fruits like ripened papaya are soft. In this way, each ingredient's qualities are to be understood.

Vipāka: After-Effects of Digestion

The change in the tastes (rasa) of a food/food ingredient that occurs at the end of digestion by the association of digestive fire is called *vipāka*. Sometimes, the vipāka taste may be different from the original taste. This is important to know because the after-effect of the taste will outlast its action on the doṣas. For example, gooseberries (amḷa) are sour in taste while eating, but sweet after digestion. This is going to help wonderfully because the sour taste helps pitta for digestion and the sweet taste balances the excess ill effects of pitta.

In general, sweet and salty tastes become sweet after digestion. Sour remains sour. The after-effect of bitter, pungent and astringent is pungent. The effect of vipāka rasa is same as pure rasa.

Conclusion

Different tastes give certain benefits to our body by aggravating or alleviating particular doṣa. So choosing the right food for you requires an understanding of rasas/tastes and they should be combined in a way that they don't counter-balance each other's benefits. Also, we need to choose the rasas that are beneficial for our particular prakṛti. One also needs cooking skills to manifest the rasa in the cooked product in a way that our body can assimilate neatly. In the following section, we will study more about the triguṇa and tridoṣa nature of food ingredients.

Section Three

Design Your Food Profile

Triguṇa and Diet
Tridoṣa of Food Ingredients
(includes Grains, Vegetables, Dairy, Oil, Spice, Fruits and Water)
Designing Your Food Profile

Design Your Food Profile

'When diet is wrong, medicine is of no use.
When diet is correct, medicine is of no need.'

—Ayurvedic Proverb

Each of us spends several years creating a unique profile for work. But we don't spend even half as much time trying to understand our bodies, food habits, what suits us and what is tough for us to digest. Each person's food profile needs to be built around their tridoṣa and triguṇa nature/prakṛti. Ideally, our work profile too needs to be built around our nature. Each person is drawn towards certain activities. Activity and appetite are interdependent. When a proper work profile is lacking in our lives, the food profile will not work for us, and the absence of a proper food profile will impact our mood, the functioning of our brain and thus our capacity to work as well. But when we are doing the right activities and consume food following pathya, or a prescribed food profile, it nourishes our nature. When our triguṇa and tridoṣa constitutions are nourished, the foundation of our health is nourished. This is described in Chart 3.1.

Chart 3.1: Cycle of Nourishment

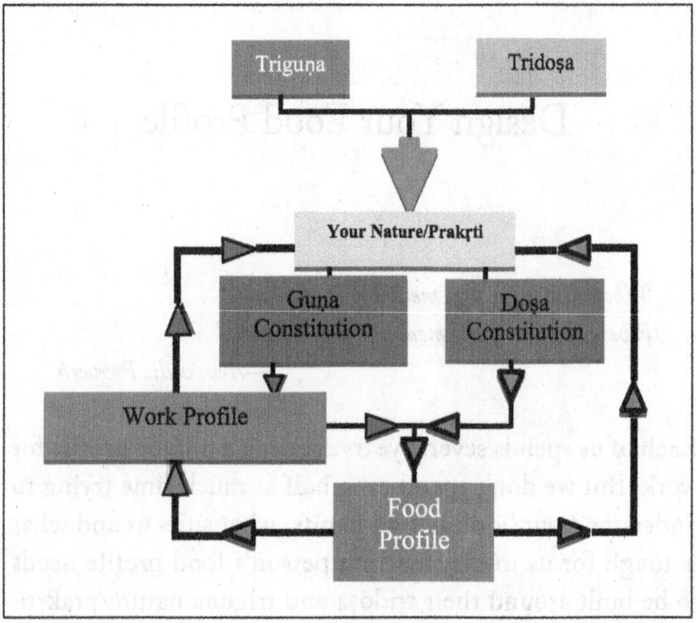

In this section, we will see how our guṇa constitution mostly decides our work profile and how our food profile needs to be attuned to our doṣa constitution. As mentioned earlier, sāttvic diet is recommended for all, irrespective of (disregarding) one's guṇa or doṣa constitution. Our tridoṣa constitution will help each of us decide which type of sāttvic food is best for us. For example, if someone is pitta prominent, they may use fenugreek seeds in their idli* batter (as it is sour and pitta increases due to fermentation), while

* Idli is made by steaming fermented batter made from a paste of soaked polished black lentils (urad dal) and rice.

those with kapha prakṛti may add some extra ginger (heating and anti-kapha) in the coconut chutney (condiment) that accompanies the idli. All these are sāttvic foods but need to be fine-tuned using the knowledge of tridoṣa. We will keep returning to this aspect.

To sketch our individual food profiles, we need to understand our tridoṣa constitution, which we did in Section One, but we also need to know the tridoṣa of the ingredients we use in our food. Two ingredients with a similar composition of fat, protein and mineral may have different triguṇa and tridoṣa constitutions: consider milk and yoghurt. Whereas cold milk (sattva guṇa) is pitta-neutralizing or cures acid refluxes, yoghurt increases it. If the yoghurt is too sour (rajo guṇa) then it further enhances pitta. So, a person having pitta constitution is advised to consume milk and not yoghurt so that it does not throw the pitta out of balance. Creating a food profile based on Ayurvedic principles goes beyond counting calories. Moreover, it's very important to see where the calories are coming from.

According to Ayurveda, a good ingredient, besides its ability to nourish the tridoṣa constitutions, is appreciated by its taste, ability to build tissue and impart prāṇa, bringing a gleam of aura called ojas (Chart 3.2). In the previous section, we discussed rasa and other properties such as hot/cool potency, the heaviness of the ingredients in terms of time required to digest, etc. All these tools along with the knowledge of tridoṣa and triguṇa will guide us to understand our individual food profiles.

Chart 3.2: Qualities of Food or Food Ingredients

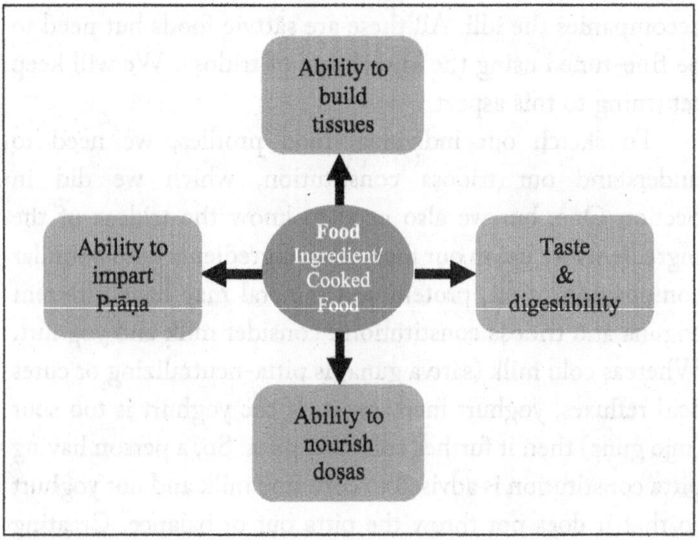

As mentioned earlier, Ayurveda also explains that a person of certain doṣa constitution should eat food that is opposite in nature to them to maintain balance and remain healthy. For example, a person of kapha prakṛti will have an affinity for sweets, which is kapha (earth element), and (an unavoidable) excess indulgence will cause obesity. So, they need to include ingredients or spices that have more pitta or fiery nature, such as pepper and ginger, to prevent excess kapha. Similarly, people of vāta prakṛti (dry and fast) need to include more oil in their diet, which is opposite in nature.

While tracking on tridoṣa nature of food, performing activities according to one's own guṇa or traits needs to be streamlined according to one's triguṇa constitution. Unfortunately, the modern competitive education system has failed to stress this important factor in guiding students. The underlying message always tends to be 'do anything' but make sure you are successful, earn well and live a comfortable life. No matter how much money and comforts one may have, one is unlikely to be happy unless the activities they perform match their inborn traits.

Years ago, I read an article about a community of farmers in Andhra Pradesh who took a loan to invest in prawn farming. They made saline water ponds out of their farmlands. They were hoping to make a fortune by exporting these prawns to the Middle East and Europe. Unfortunately, the plan backfired and not only did the fish not take to the habitat, but the farmlands were also rendered infertile as they had been flooded with saltwater. They were left with no means to repay the bank loan. Many of them committed suicide. The community tried to emulate a model that had been successful for certain other entrepreneurs.

People inclined towards business are endowed with the mental capacity to bear losses and start a new business to succeed. During Partition, many business people left all their property and businesses in Pakistan and fled to India, and vice versa. They started from scratch in their new cities. No doubt what they went through was deeply traumatic, but because they were empowered by mother nature with the trait of tolerance for loss in business, most of them gradually became successful again. The farmers, however, had an aptitude and taste for farming and not business. Similarly, people are inclined to be artists, thinkers, scientists, administrators, architects, etc. One should follow one's own trait and not try to become someone else. A relaxed and satisfied mind contributes significantly to healthy digestion. We will discuss this further in the digestion section.

Irrespective of how circumstances shape one's career, the guṇa or inborn qualities keep propelling us towards certain activities. For example, one may be an engineer by education, but one may choose to teach engineering rather than work as an engineer. It is wise to recognize and listen to these inner callings. One may earn less money as a professor, but one will be more happy and satisfied.

Triguṇa and Diet

As mentioned earlier, Ayurveda and yoga literature recommends a sāttvic diet or food in the mode of goodness, irrespective of which guṇa one may belong to. A sāttvic diet, by constitution, is preserving and balancing. It enhances the positive aspects of people of all guṇa constitutions and empowers them to regulate and curtail negative impacts of passion and ignorance. Staying in one's own nature means focusing on the brighter side of that nature and curtailing or regulating the darker side. A sāttvic diet helps one grow without stepping out of one's own nature. Without such help, the negative aspects of the rajo and tama guṇa will throttle one's growth. For example, if we let go of the steering wheel while driving, the car will run itself off the road. Similarly, the negative attributes of passion and ignorance weigh us down and push us off the path of the good life. Therefore, one needs to nourish a sāttvic nature through diet and other sāttvic activities to get the best of the triguṇa nature that one is blessed with. But that doesn't mean everyone will have to eat the same food. No, adjustments must be made according to tridoṣa nature, activities, place and climate, etc., before deciding on the final food profile. For example, a person living in Kashmir (northern India) will have a different sāttvic diet from one living in Kanyakumari (southern India). Let's try to understand how sāttvic food is different from rājasic and tāmasic food.

Sāttvic Food: Food for Thought!

āyuḥ-sattva-balārogya-
sukha-prīti-vivardhanāḥ
rasyāḥ snigdhāḥ sthirā hṛdyā
āhārāḥ sāttvika-priyāḥ

—Bhagavad Gitā 17.8

Foods dear to those in the mode of goodness increase the duration of life (āyuḥ), purify one's existence and give strength (*bala*), diseaseless body (ārogya) and increased health, happiness and satisfaction. Such foods are juicy, fatty, wholesome, and pleasing to the heart (*sthirā hṛdyā*).

Food and Mind: Bhagavad Gitā, a life-treatise revealed by Lord Krishna out of affection for his dear friend Arjuna, enumerates all the 'pure' qualities of sāttvic food in a nutshell. Ayurveda is all about longevity. But what is the use of a long life without peace, happiness and satisfaction? Contrarily, a long life is not possible without these qualities. So, naturally, Ayurveda emphasizes a sāttvic diet that not only imparts longevity, but also keeps one's mind clear, content and happy. Sāttvic food has a direct positive impact on the mind and creates a deep sense of satisfaction (ātma santusṭi) at the end of a meal.

The main purpose of sāttvic diet, however, is to develop higher consciousness. One turns inward, with a desire to know the self and the world's intricacies, when the mind is calm and not restless. Such enquiries give further satisfaction, and with an empowered, steady and sharp mind, one is able to gradually find answers to life's pressing questions. Such people, free from anxieties and enlightened with knowledge, become truly selfless and engage only to benefit others. This is perfectly described in the Chāndogya Upaniṣad (Chart 3.3).

āhāra suddhau sattva suddḥi
sattva-suddhau dhruva smṛtiḥ
dhruva smṛti lambhe
sarva granthinaṁ vipra mokṣḥ

—Chāndogya Upaniṣad 7.26.2

Yogis and saints who meditate for long hours often recognize the strong link between food and the mind, and are very careful about the food they eat. Food, according to the Ayurveda and Yoga philosophy, should nourish the body, which is made up of doṣas, and the mind, which is made up of guṇas. Sāttvic food nourishes and maintains the balance of tridoṣa, nourishes sattva guṇa, keeps rajas and tamas in check and nourishes the mind by bringing satisfaction. According to the teaching of the Gitā, it's very difficult to keep our mind satisfied. Indeed, satisfaction is mentioned to be an austerity for the mind!

Modern-day nutritionists focus only on physical health—muscles, tissues, heart, pancreas, blood sugar, gut flora, thyroid glands, skin and hair, joints, bones, lungs, etc. They are unable to link food to the mind or beyond. But a true practitioner of yoga is more concerned with mental health. Because a strong healthy mind can endure physical pain, but not vice versa. If the mind is weak, even a minor physical ailment can cause a lot of worry.

How to Classify an Ingredient as Sāttvic

An ingredient is classified as sattva, rajas or tamas depending on the impact it has on the body and mind. If it induces sattva, then the ingredient is classified as sāttvic. But how does one determine this? Different sources vary on what is sāttvic. Let us consider a few examples to understand this.

Onion and Garlic: One source I checked classified onion as sāttvic, whereas ancient texts consider it tāmasic. So much so that in some Devi temples, where animals are sacrificed, onion and garlic are not used to cook the sacrificial meat as these two ingredients will 'contaminate' the meat. So, who should we listen to? Ayurveda and Yoga are ancient sciences and were a result of many saintly personalities studying the nature of the ingredients, and using their knowledge to classify them. Thus, it is best to follow credible sources. Dr J.V. Hebbar, currently an Ayurvedic lecturer and a popular author and blogger (easyayurveda.com), classifies onion as tāmasic. Dr Robert E. Svoboda, a prolific author and Ayurvedic doctor, says that garlic and onions are both rājasic and tāmasic, forbidden to yogis because they root the consciousness more firmly in the body. All the traditional yoga masters such as Swami Sivananda, Swami Paramahansa Yogananda and Maharshi Mahesh Yogi, adhering to a sāttvic diet, do not eat onion and garlic. Sripada Ramanujācārya, and in recent years Srila Bhakti Vedanta Swami Prabhupada, who are authorities on Vaishnava culture, classify onions and garlic as tāmasic.

Ayurveda says that apart from producing bad breath and body odour, allium plants (onion, garlic, chives and leek) induce aggravation, agitation, anxiety and aggression. Thus, they can be harmful physically, emotionally (mentally) and spiritually. So, onion is classified by many as rājasic and to some extent as tāmasic.

Modern scientific research reveals that both onion and garlic contain sulphoxide (a compound that contains sulfinyl (SO) functional group attached to two carbon atoms). Sulphoxide increases blood flow, which in turn influences the muscles and the brain (resulting in agitation). However, garlic, for this very reason, is good for people who suffer from high blood pressure and cardiac constrictions. Both onion and garlic belong to the genus allium, which includes shallot, leek and chives. The chemicals in these plants can cause severe irritation, kill microbes and repel insects. Both onion and garlic are classified as FODMAP (Fermentable Oligo-, Di-, Mono-saccharides and Polyols) by modern dieticians, known to cause irritable bowel syndrome and other gut symptoms. Because FODMAPs are short chains of sugars, they are 'osmotically active'. This means they pull water from your body tissue into your intestine (For example, when you eat the FODMAP fructose, it draws twice as much water into your intestine as glucose, which is not a FODMAP). This can lead to symptoms such as bloating and diarrhea for people who have sensitive digestive systems.

So, in conclusion, Ayurveda doesn't prohibit consumption of onion or garlic (or for that matter meat products), as long as there are health benefits. But it doesn't recommend eating them at every meal as it would do with any other medicine. However, Ayurveda does classify them as tāmasic and thus are not healthy in ultimate terms as, apart from breath, the purity of the mind would also be compromised.

Rice and Millet: Let's take two more examples. It is said that people involved in jobs that require higher mental and intellectual engagement should eat rice, which is sāttvic, because it is easy to digest and adds to the mental faculties. Millets, on the other hand, are recommended for people who must do hard labour through the day, such as farmers. Millets improve physical strength and are also easy to digest, thus providing an instant source of sustained energy. As millets increase only bodily strength, they are categorized as rājasic. Millets are considered a superfood in many parts of the world and pesticides and genetic modification have not completely changed this category of food. But the quality of rice and wheat, which is more popular, has been severely impacted by genetic engineering and chemical fertilizers.

What Makes an Ingredient Sāttvic?

Now, in this era of globalization, when so many new ingredients flood our kitchens, it might be tougher to classify them under sattva, rajas and tamas. Some ingredients are easy to recognize. For example, if it is a fermented product and causes drowsiness, it is in the category of tamas. If something agitates or stimulates our senses or creates a lot of heat in the body, it may be categorized as rājasic. Ingredients that do not disturb the doṣas or the mind much can be classified as sāttvic.

Fresh Food: Fresh ripe fruits and freshly cooked food from fresh vegetables and grains are some examples of sāttvic food. Freshness contributes to the sāttvic nature of an ingredient. Think of it this way—only life can sustain life. Fresh food has life. Apart from protein, fat and minerals, Ayurveda speaks about the potency or prāṇa-śakti of food. Prāṇa means vitality or life, and śakti means force or energy. Prāṇa refers to life-force. This is primarily found in food, water and the air we breathe. Pure fresh food, clean spring water and fresh forest air have maximum prāṇa. When we cut off a branch from a tree, it lives for some time and then gradually withers and dies. Similarly, fresh fruits, vegetables and salad, plucked from a living plant, have maximum prāṇa. Grains, even if aged, have life, because when planted, these germinate into saplings.

Animals, like cows who have four stomachs, can digest all types of raw food, including grains. But humans need to cook grains with water and fire to make them fit for digestion. So, freshly cooked grains have more prāṇa. Cooked food, with time, starts to go bad and loose prāṇa-śakti. Therefore, frozen foods have very little prāṇa, although such food may still have the protein, fat and mineral quantities intact, as well as the taste. However, one can clearly feel the difference in energy levels while consuming food with high prāṇic quotient.

When Does Sāttvic Food Turn Rājasic/Tāmasic?

It's important to note here that the cooking method and the cook's mentality matters a lot while cooking sāttvic food. For example, if we add too much salt or spices to sāttvic ingredients, the final product will be rājasic and not sāttvic. Similarly, if the food is overcooked or gets burnt, it becomes tāmasic. A positive mental attitude of care and love while cooking adds to the sāttvic quality of the food. On the other hand, a desire to gain prominence (as a chef) lends the food a rājasic nature, while an attitude of envy and hatred makes the food tāmasic even if the ingredients are sāttvic. Keeping something pure is always challenging but satisfying at the end. So, cooking sāttvic food is quite a challenge and requires a good deal of training and practice. We will explore this further in the next section while discussing cooking procedures.

Variety: Somehow, a myth persists that sāttvic food is bland and bereft of good taste, that it is meant for sick people, and so on. But the reality is that sāttvic food is full of variety, and its ingredients can be combined in many ways to provide taste, good health and satisfaction. I have been eating and feeding sāttvic food for twenty-five years now and trust me, I am not bored with it. Even today, a lot of sāttvic food is cooked in the homes of millions of families all over the world, on festive days.

Sometime ago, a friend of mine organized an international yoga camp in Rishikesh, India. Yoga guru Sharath Jois was invited to conduct the sessions, and I was honoured with the service of cooking for the students for a week or so. There were about 200 students, who had come from all over the world to attend the camp. We cooked pure sāttvic food from locally available, fresh ingredients. I was surprised that everyone liked and appreciated the food, and there wasn't a single complaint! Initially, I thought it would be very challenging to satisfy the taste buds of people from Japan, Iran, Mexico, Indonesia,

China, the US, Russia, the UK and many other countries with the same meal. Of course, we made adjustments for a few people who had specific health issues arising from jet lag and a change in the climate. That camp made me realize the power of sāttvic food.

While preparing sāttvic food, the spices and ingredients are cooked in a way that does not disturb the tridoṣa balance. In Section Five, you will find some recipes along with an explanation on the use of ingredients and spices for various tridoṣic prakṛti.

Table 3.1 and 3.2 summarize the details of sāttvic food. In conclusion, the food ingredients that are preserving, easy to digest, increase memory and promote positive thinking are sāttvic, the food ingredients which agitate the senses, create heat in the body and cause sexual desire and greed are rājasic. Those that cause lethargy and negative thinking are tāmasic.

Table 3.1: Food Ingredients in Different Guṇas (Examples)

Ingredients	Sāttvic Food	Rājasic Food*	Tāmasic Food
Grains	Rice, barley, sago, amaranth	Millets, yellow corn, buckwheat	Fermented grains to produce alcoholic drinks
Vegetables	Fresh vegetables: ridge gourd, yellow squash, sweet potatoes, zucchini, triphalā, leafy vegetables, sprouts	Potatoes, tomatoes, cauliflower, pickles, tea	Mushrooms, onion, garlic, chives, tobacco

* Some of these ingredients, like salt, are also used in sāttvic cooking, but when the use is in excess, then it turns to rājasic.

Ingredients	**Sāttvic Food**	**Rājasic Food**	**Tāmasic Food**
Fruits	Coconut, pomegranate, apple, guava, figs, peaches, pears, mango	Sharp citrus fruits, e.g. tamarind, dates, papaya	Fermented fruits or wine, vinegar
Beans/ Legumes	Green moong, white beans, pigeon pea lentils	Rajma/red kidney beans, coffee, cocoa	Red lentils, black lentils
Dairy	Cow milk, fresh yoghurt, buttermilk, fresh cream, fresh cottage cheese, fresh mozzarella	Sour yoghurt, sour cream	Buffalo milk, aged cheese, all processed products—butter, yoghurt etc
Spices and Herbs	Cumin, coriander, mustard, fennel, turmeric, fenugreek, cinnamon, bay leaf, ginger, saffron, cilantro, mint, basil, sage, unbleached sea/Himalayan salt, rosemary, curry leaf, amalaki, cardamom	Salt, chilli peppers. asafoetida, clove	Overcooked and burnt spices. Use of wine and similar beverages in cooking
Others	Organic products of honey, jaggery, raw sugar, nuts, herbal tea	Chocolates, black tea, refined sugar, white flour	All meat products, frozen/ chemically preserved food

Table 3.2: Impact of Food on Gross and Subtle Body

Triguṇa Impact	Sāttvic Food	Rājasic Food	Tāmasic Food
on Body	Gains strength, vigour, vitality	Misery while eating and sickness afterwards	Weakens body and joints, lethargy
on Doṣa	All three doṣas get nourished and stay in balance*	Pitta goes out of balance and then vāta or kapha or both	All three doṣas get disturbed
on Mind	Satisfaction, peaceful, focused, selfless work	Greed, anger, self-centred thoughts	Depression, frustration, passive for constructive work and active for (self) destructive work.
on Self	Desire for philosophical knowledge	Desire for material opulence	Unhealthy desire for material opulence
Recommendation	Every morsel	Occasionally under guidance	Under strict supervision

* This depends upon the individual doṣas. The sāttvic food needs to match the doṣa constitution.

Rājasic Food: Food for the senses!

kaṭv-amla-lavaṇāty-uṣṇa-
tīkṣṇa-rūkṣa-vidāhinaḥ
āhārā rājasasyeṣṭā
duḥkha-śokāmaya-pradāḥ

—Bhagavad Gitā 17.9

Foods that are too bitter, too sour, salty, hot, pungent, dry and burning are dear to those in the mode of passion. Such foods cause distress, misery and disease.

Food Is Our Friend: Rājasic food is designed to provide intense pleasure, and the health aspect takes a back seat with such food. As mentioned earlier, the word Rājā means king and denotes enjoyment. A king, a true warrior, doesn't enjoy a fight unless the opponent is a good match and lands him a couple of good punches. Similarly, food in the mode of passion draws one to relish it to the point of pain. Anything extreme is rājasic. The senses are stimulated when there is a sensation of pinching or hurt. But food should always be our friend and not our enemy. Like a passionate king who needs a saintly mentor, food can always be sāttvic.

Immediate Effect and Long-Term Effect: Eating rājasic food almost brings about a sense of misery. For example, excess chilli pepper brings tears to the eyes and causes one to sweat. Later, it causes distress in the digestive tract. It hurts while eating and it burns while passing. If consumed on a regular basis, it causes chronic sickness. Despite this, those who are rājasic/passionate by nature will develop a longing for such food. Take another example—potato chips. Most commercially produced chips contain a lot of excess salt. One is unable to stop eating till the last tiny piece is consumed. I've seen people eat spicy food the same way too. Such food disturbs the pitta doṣa for sure and thus adversely affects the balance of vāta and kapha. Although people with rājasic nature will be drawn to such food, Ayurveda advises they should not indulge in such food and promote their passionate side.

Sāttvic food, on the other hand, will help a person of rājasic nature utilize their passionate ability to rule or lead better. To derive the same amount of satisfaction, they can increase the proportion of protein in their sāttvic meals.

Impact on Mental Strength: While sāttvic food has a positive impact on mental health, rājasic food is designed to agitate the senses and mind. This unfortunately leads to hankering for more, resulting in greed. This results in two types of anxieties, to preserve what one has and to grow more. Such anxieties are likely to affect sleep and alter blood pressure. And this in turn affects digestion and appetite. When one is not hungry, the only food they reach for is that which is appealing to or shocks the senses. That is rājasic food. Thus, one falls into a vicious cycle, which can result in chronic problems arising out of imbalances of doṣas, such as obesity and high blood pressure.

Can I Eat Rājasic Food at All?

One may ask, why does such food exist at all, then? There is always a good reason for the existence of every creation. For example, during pregnancy, mothers-to-be hanker for tangy food, like pickles, and dry snacks like puffed rice. In some parts of India, the custom is for daughters to send a letter to their mothers requesting pickle to indirectly inform them of their pregnancy.

During pregnancy, the amount of amniotic fluid in the body increases. As a result, the haemoglobin content is diluted, a phenomenon known as haemo-dilution. The lack of haemoglobin creates a craving for sour preparations (*Astānga*

Hṛdayam, Sutra Sthana 11.173*). Pickles that are sun-dried and prepared using traditional recipes are preferred. But pickle doesn't replenish haemoglobin. That is possible only through proper medication and other dietary supplements. Pickle simply curbs the hankering and should not be consumed in excess. Sāttvic food keeps the doṣas of the mother as well as the developing child in balance.

So, as a king needs to follow the guidance of ministers, one needs to consume rājasic food under the guidance of a wise doctor or dietician. While occasional consumption will not create any issues, frequent consumption is not recommended.

Tāmasic Food: Food for destruction

yāta-yāmaṁ gata-rasaṁ
pūti paryuṣitaṁ ca yat
ucchiṣṭam api cāmedhyaṁ
bhojanaṁ tāmasa-priyam

—Bhagavad Gitā 17.9

Food prepared more than three hours before being eaten, food that is tasteless, decomposed and putrid, and food consisting of remnants and untouchable things (liquor, flesh, blood and bones, rotten food) is dear to those in the mode of darkness.

* *Rakte* (in lack of blood), amḷa (sour), *śiśir* (cold), *priti* (liking), *śira-śouthilya rukṣhatā*
Decrease in rakta-dhātu (haemoglobin) causes dryness in skin, desire towards sour and cold food substances and flaccidity in the veins.
—*Astānga Hṛdayam, Sutra Sthana 11.17*

Danger Zone: Tamas means ignorance, callousness towards distress. Tāmasic food, which is generally stale and fermented food, causes stubborn inertia, inertness and laziness, which can potentially lead to depression. This is due to lack of prāṇa or life force in such food, as it is not fresh. Even sāttvic food, in a very strict sense, becomes tāmasic after three hours of cooking. But in the modern-day scenario, it seems impossible to have fresh food for every meal. The next best thing we can adopt is to keep the food out of the 'danger zone'. Because in this zone, the harmful bacteria become active and make food unfit for consumption. This danger zone is in the temperature range of 5–58°Celsius (41–136°F). According to ISO 22000, food that is left unattended in this 'danger zone' for four hours is unfit to consume. Nowadays, slow cookers cook food slowly and keep it hot for a long time. The second best thing is to cool down the food to room temperature and refrigerate it below 5° Celsius (41°F). In that way, at least the harmful bacteria will be kept at bay. Following these principles, if we overeat sāttvic food and if it is not digested in three or four hours, it turns tāmasic in our stomach and becomes harmful for the same reason. So, ISO recommends that one stores cooked food below 5 or above 55°C. However, Ayurveda doesn't consider that to be the best practice either. Overheating/overcooking or reheating refrigerated food will disturb the prāṇa-śakti (life force) of the food that freshly cooked food offers. When we cook food, we basically bring unripe, raw ingredients to a ripe digestible stage. Just as one can't re-ripen or further ripen an already ripened fruit, we can't reheat or overcook already cooked food. To the extent, Ayurveda considers reheating drinking water that is already boiled once to be poisonous. All being said, note that certain dry items like puffed rice, flat chipped rice (pohā), roasted nuts and lentils or fried nuts and lentils can be stored for long at normal temperature in an airtight container. This point will be elaborated later on in this section.

Lifeless Food: Apart from sāttvic and rājasic food that is three to four hours old, burnt food, even if it is freshly cooked from sāttvic ingredients, is considered tāmasic. So is food that is very dry, without any rasa or juice (gata rasaṁ). All chemically preserved packaged foods and frozen foods are also tāmasic, because the life force is altered or affected. These types of foods are very likely to push all the three tridoṣa body constitution out of balance, thus inviting sickness. Tāmasic food lowers the body's ability to fight disease and disrupts the proper functioning of the immune system because of its intoxicating effects. The good thing about sāttvic food is that everyone likes it. So when a tāmasic person consumes sāttvic food, their health will improve, and slowly they will emerge from the inertia and be engaged. But sometimes our nature may rule over the mind, and a craving for a particular type of food may arise. In such scenarios, one should consume such food with regulation and care, and not get addicted.

Impact on Mental Strength: I read the manual for driving for California State and was especially amazed to read the section on how strictly they deal with drivers under the influence (DUI) of alcohol or drugs. A first offense, for example, is a misdemeanour typically punished by three to five years of probation, $390 to $1000 in fines plus penalty assessments, DUI school course, a six-month driver's licence suspension, and installation of an ignition interlock device (IID).

The IID basically doesn't allow the car engine to start if it detects alcohol on the driver's breath. The mind and the intelligence both are adversely affected by such food and drinks. They can drive a person to a negative state of mind, which in turn can encourage telling lies, stealing money, etc. and push one to activities that facilitate depression and destructive behaviour.

Is Fresh Meat Sāttvic?

Does all fresh food qualify as sāttvic? The answer is no. Meat is a product of violence. Eating meat is considered tāmasic as one is callous to the pain of the dying animal. Many people refuse to eat meat if they see an animal being slaughtered, at least for some time. An Ayurvedic diet, however, does not exclude meat, because certain people cannot live without meat. Since Ayurveda is meant to preserve human life in the first place, it does allow for the consumption of certain animal flesh. Raw meat and similar produce spoils very quickly, and can create a host of issues. There are strict modern regulations for handling meat products in groceries and restaurants serving such products. Ayurveda explains how to process, cook and consume meat in a way that is good for human health.

Another valid reason for meat consumption is lack of vegetation in places such as Antarctica and deserts.

Food As Medicine

You may wonder, does tāmasic food have any utility at all? Yes, it can treat some ailments. Ayurveda recommends the use of home-made alcohol (asava) to treat ailments, such as fever, cough and cold. Some tāmasic food helps you rest well and numbs the senses during sickness.

In Odisha, the state I come from, it's a standard practice to soak cooked rice in water overnight, especially during summer. It is eaten with yoghurt and green chillis to beat the heat of summer. It is sometimes eaten with baked vegetables or pakoras. Such food naturally slows down the body and mind, allowing one to rest well. This is tāmasic, yet useful to beat the heat of summer. But considering the intoxicating effect of such food, one is advised to consume it only under guidance.

Conclusion

At this point, I'm sure you must be wondering, should I switch over to a sāttvic diet? The answer is yes. But the shift must be gradual. At times it can be challenging, but overall, it will be enjoyable. There will be an immediate increase in your mental peace and good health, but the real transformation takes time. Just as rājasic food can lead to chronic diseases over time, sāttvic food takes time to recover any good health that is lost. It may take less time to heal the effects of rājasic food than tāmasic food. Nature works in small installments, just as a baby that develops in the womb, slow and steady. One needs patience and perseverance through the process.

Transformation does not mean changing one's tridoṣa, triguṇa and karma (activities),* rather it means revitalizing your original nature from a troubled state. It means to revive from a sick state to normal state of nature.

* Bhagavad Gitā 3.35 and 18.47

Diet and Tridoṣa

I lived in the ashram of Sri Sri Radha Gopinath Mandir of ISKCON in Mumbai as a monk for more than twenty years. I was one among 250 other monks. We led a sāttvic lifestyle and always ate sāttvic food while living in the ashram. We never ate in restaurants, except on very rare occasions, in Govindas, our temple restaurant, which serves sāttvic prasādam. Even while going on holy trips, we ate only sāttvic food, either from some ashrams, or cooked on our own.

I was head chef for the ashram for over ten years and would cook for all the ashram inmates as well as the serving staff. During annual festivals and holy pilgrimages to places like Vrindavan, I would lead the cooking for nearly 6000 members continuously for nearly two weeks and serve about 10,000 plates of sāttvic meals per day.

Despite the sincere effort to provide sāttvic food, I observed that some of the people living in the ashram would face health issues. So, as the head chef of the ashram, I was concerned, and pondered deeply. Sometimes, people would receive packages from their homes and offer it to me. I would be delighted to try. Sometimes, people would offer me the food as a subtle hint that this is how they wanted the food in the ashram to taste every day. Sometimes I would find that the home food was extremely spicy or bland. Occasionally, it would not suit me. Each household cooks according to the particular nature/taste they are accustomed to. That is when I realized that the sāttvic food I was cooking needed to be fine-tuned to match the prakṛti of each person eating the meal. Besides, each monk had developed different unique sātmya from the food habits they have been subjected to.

But since there were over 200 of us, from all over India, it was not practical to cater to individual needs. Instead, we planned two separate menus with multiple choices, so that people could pick best according to their doṣas and nature. This slight change to provide the right choices had an excellent impact and reduced health issues by nearly 80 per cent.

That is when I learnt that the best person to understand the prakṛti of a person is the cook in their household. Fine-tuning your diet to your tridoṣa is much easier within a family. This is probably why in India, many wandering saints/sādhus always insist on cooking their own food. This is particularly of relevance to frequent travellers as well. If possible, one should make sure to eat from the hands of the same caring cook as much as possible. Otherwise, Ayurveda warns that travelling too much makes a young man old.

The same elements that build up our body also form the food ingredients that nourish our body. From all that we've touched upon so far, it must be clear that depending on our body's tridoṣa constitution, certain food ingredients are good for us while others are not.

For example, as a child I used to fall ill if I would have pani poori. Pani poori is a crispy puffed salty pastry stuffed with mashed potatoes and peas, and filled with spicy, sweet and sour water. The whole stuffed poori has to be eaten at one go, leading to an explosion of rasās or tastes of various ingredients within the mouth.

My friend, Dr Sanjay, an Ayurvedic doctor who inspired me to write this book, had analysed my tridoṣa prakṛti as pitta-kapha. This helped me understand why pani poori and similar food does not suit me. The acidic nature of the sour tamarind in pani poori would aggravate my pitta doṣa, while the cold pani would aggravate my kapha doṣa. Aggravated kapha reduces the digestive fire and this in turn puts pitta doṣa further out of balance. The result is acid reflux and indigestion. I was a bit disappointed to learn this because I love eating pani poori. But it also shows us that there is an uncanny attraction towards food that is opposite to our nature. So, it is important to keep such cravings in check.

Pitta doṣa becomes more prominent during youth. So people with pitta constitutions, especially when they are young, need to be vigilant of ingredients that may aggravate pitta doṣa. So understanding the nature of food ingredient can help us avoid issues. One of my ashram inmates once invited me to his parents' home in Pune. After over an hour or so of having a full Marwari meal, his sister came with pani poori. She runs a pani poori shop in Pune and wanted me to try some of those. I was already full and as such pani poori gives me trouble. So I was in a tight spot, but just to please her, I agreed. As expected, I just could not stop eating the pani poori. It was perfect and delicious. It was a rainy afternoon and as we drove back to Mumbai, I was wondering what suffering awaited me. But I had a surprisingly smooth passage. I called my friend in Pune and asked how the pani had been made. I discovered that his sister uses amḷa (gooseberries) instead of imli (tamarind) as a souring agent among other Ayurvedic herbs. I was amazed how changing one critical ingredient could completely change my experience with a dish that usually caused me a lot of trouble.

So, apart from understanding our nature, it is important that we learn the nature of food ingredients. Understanding food ingredients and products in terms of tridoṣa will help us design our food profile more precisely. Table 3.3 gives a broad classification of tridoṣa of different ingredients and its impact on our body. However, before we discuss the doṣa of food ingredients, it's important to know how pure the ingredients you are cooking with are. Here we will discuss two aspects of ingredients in the following order.

Table 3.3: Food Ingredients and Doṣa

Tridoṣa	Helpful for	Example of Food Ingredients
Kapha	Building tissues, muscles and bones	Rice, vegetables
Vāta	Movement, activity, transportation within the body	Legumes, beans, dairy products
Pitta	Digestion, body temperature	Ginger, pepper, chilli

Purity of Food Ingredients

> *Don't ask why healthy food is so expensive. Ask why junk food is so cheap.*
>
> —*Nutrition Snob*

Organic Food: In this age of biotechnology, it's difficult to find ingredients in their original forms. Just as a woman gives birth to a beautiful baby and creates food for the baby in the form of her milk, mother nature gives birth to all kinds of living entities and takes care of their food too. So, if we change the genetic structure of the food supplied by nature according to our convenience, it will not be in perfect harmony with our bodies, which in turn is likely to create health issues.

There is a harmony between the structure of food supplied by nature and our own genes. So, when we modify the food through biotechnology, which is popularly known as GMO (genetically modified organism) food, this harmony is disrupted. Most of the modifications are to protect and promote commercial interests than promoting health benefits. For example, I remember that the tomatoes I used to buy thirty years ago used to have a very thin skin. But the newer varieties available now are larger and thick-skinned. They have been modified this way to minimize losses during transportation and maximize profit. But the flipside is that these are not as easy to digest. A *New York Times* article on 15 April 1975 reported as follows:

'Over the last few years the tomato has become a symbol for consumer groups of everything they find wrong with the American food supply. Today's supermarket tomato is a thick-skinned mutant of its former juicy self, designed to be mass grown, mass shipped and mass marketed.'

The article went on to report that people are disappointed with the taste and flavour of the mutated tomatoes. And after sometime when this generation of people leaves the planet, nobody will remain to talk about the good old days.

While there is widespread research pointing that genetically mutated/modified agricultural produce is safe, the WHO keeps a strict vigil on research for editing the human genome. I find it strange that the same organization promotes the idea that GMO food is safe.

With the advent of globalization, people have begun to grow produce in soils and climates that are not indigenous to the produce. This is yet another reason why pesticides are required. For example, vegetables that grow in a dry cold climate do not have protective thick skin like those that grow in warm humid weather. Bacteria and other organisms grow and thrive in a warm, humid climate. When we try to grow vegetables that grow well in dry, cold weather, such as cauliflower, cabbage and capsicum in a warm climate, pesticides are required in larger proportions. This is because unlike pumpkins (bhopla/kaddu) and bottle gourd (lauki/doodhi), there is no natural thick skin on such vegetables to protect them. For example, the level of pesticides in capsicum (bell peppers) in India is thirty to forty times higher than that in Europe where the climate is cool and dry. So, even when we travel, we should only look for food prepared from local ingredients, and which suit our prakṛti or nature. Now, genetically corrected capsicums have thick skin and they may claim it requires less pesticides, but the thick skin will have an impact on our digestion. We just need to think soberly.

Some of my childhood was spent in a remote village. I remember eating simple food cooked from fresh, organic produce. The taste of that pure food is deeply imprinted in my mind. But sadly, we have moved far away from such ingredients. One thing that I know for sure is that the advent of chemical fertilizers and GMO food has had a telling impact on the taste of food ingredients. It is time that we return those vehicles of good health to our future generations. If you have a small garden or a terrace space, do try some farming. Grow some fruits and vegetables. You will be amazed by the taste and freshness of the organic food. And if possible, grow some grains. A family of four needs just an acre of land to grow all the food they need throughout the year. Kristen Satre Meyer, an environmental journalist, says that a vegetarian requires only 0.35 acres of land for sustenance.*

Fifteen years ago, I met the father of one of my students in a remote village in India. He was around fifty-six years old. Every day, he would walk barefoot for at least eight kilometres to look after his farm. Most of the monthly expenditure was only for kerosene to help ignite the wood for cooking and burn a lamp at night, as they couldn't rely on the erratic power supply.

They were healthy and happy with their lives. In the evening, we sat together, and I read from the Bhagavad Gitā under the glow of a lantern. They enjoyed the tenets on peace and contentment in the Gitā, and I realized that they were truly practising it in their lives, living in harmony with nature.

Simple living gradually takes one inward and brings inner peace and calm. A clear mind is key to good health and happiness. Farming is an activity that naturally encourages slowing down and connecting with nature. You need not own large pieces of land to benefit from the soothing act of planting seeds, nurturing them and watching them grow and produce fresh food. You can grow herbs and vegetables in pots, wherever you live.

To conclude, if the ingredients are not pure, then the subtle and refined principles of Ayurveda cannot help much.

Factory-Processed Food

Ayurvedic principles outline that some dry food can be stored and consumed, especially while travelling. Lack of moisture protects the food for days and it does not turn tāmasic.

* https://ensia.com/notable/which-diet-makes-best-use-of-farmland-you-might-be-surprised/

Roasted nuts, puffed rice and roasted flat rice fall into this category, and can be stored in airtight containers for up to three weeks. Usually, such food is served with a dash of cold-pressed oil, fresh lemon juice and with easily digestible raw vegetables, such as cucumber. Such preparations are called bhel, jhal muri, etc, across different parts of India. But similar products that are processed and packaged in factories often contain chemicals to preserve the food. These chemicals/preservatives are produced artificially.

But why does packaged food have chemicals in it, you may ask? That's because factories produce all the products in very large quantities, much more than shops can sell before the food spoils. In some cases, it takes longer than that time just to reach the shops. It could be a few months before the consumer eats the food. So, the producers are forced to add preservatives that prevent the food from spoiling. Consequently, the prāṇa/vitality in such food is very low.

The preservatives prevent other organisms from eating the food. In other words, these chemicals are anti-life. Not only do the preservatives kill the microorganisms, but they are also unfit for consumption. This is because the preservatives continue to preserve the food in our stomach, preventing digestion. Our stomach, which is like a second brain with an independent nervous system that can operate without any assistance from the brain or spinal cord, disregards these chemicals as they do not form a part of the natural food cycle, and as a result, digestion is affected. These substances also affect the natural healthy flora culture in our gut, which can lead to acid reflux and similar digestive problems. But producers are aware of this also and add an acidity regulator to the preserved processed food to manage indigestions caused by the preservatives. To make the food more appealing, some also add more chemicals such as taste enhancers and food colouring.

Apart from all these artificial chemicals that the body does not know how to digest, such food has low prāṇa.

Our body is very sophisticated, and the food we feed it needs to be very pure. Just as a car that runs on petrol cannot run on diesel, the body needs fuel that is perfectly attuned to its inner working.

Anything that enters our digestive canal that is not found in the natural food cycle may be rejected by the body. The digestive tract is like a canal or river. All the useful things that are transported through this river enter our body during the digestive process. But note that the mouth is not the gateway to our body. Rather, it is the stomach. Our body grows around the alimentary canal, like a civilization grows around a river. If this river or canal is not kept free from pollutants, it will be very difficult to enjoy good health.

Thus, it is better to stay away from processed food and preservatives as much as possible. Pure, fresh ingredients are more than capable of nourishing us and can also be prepared in a way that helps us relish the food.

We need to return to older and time-tested ways of growing and cooking our food. We need to keep away from the methods that modify our food so radically that it potentially harms the human body.

Unless we make it a habit to procure fresh organic food ingredients, we can't expect to fully benefit from practising the Ayurvedic principles of cooking food. When Ayurvedic principles linked to food were formulated, ingredients and methods of processing were very different. The industrial revolution was yet to happen.

Tridoṣa of Food Ingredients

Each ingredient is a combination of certain doṣas, irrespective of the fat, protein and mineral content. We discussed how two different ingredients may have the same calorific values but have different doṣa qualities. It is the doṣas that determine what is suitable for a person and how the calories are used up by the body. Sometimes the doṣa of a particular ingredient can be moderated through the method of cooking. It's important to note here that we cannot moderate or reduce the impact of chemicals and genetic modification used in agriculture through cooking. In this discussion, we will choose some of the most commonly used ingredients and classify them according to their doṣa.

How Will Tridoṣa Information about the Food Ingredients Help You?

It's an everyday struggle to keep our constitutional doṣa nature in balance. We may be perfectly fine in the morning, and feel off colour by the evening. Our doṣa could go out of balance for so many reasons, and while keeping track of one factor, we may lose sight of another. A chilly and windy winter morning can disturb our kapha while a late night dinner or a movie can throw our pitta off balance. Like steering a car on a highway, if we are not vigilant, we will go off track. But what do we do if we do steer out of our lane? We correct course before an accident occurs. Either by adjusting diet or by fasting, or by performing yoga āsanas, prāṇāyāma, kriyās (cleansing processes) or by resting, we can bring the doṣas back to equilibrium and prevent diseases. So, having some knowledge of ingredients helps a lot to preserve doṣa balance.

For example, if an imbalance in pitta is causing acid reflux, we should drink water, fresh lemon juice with misri (sugar candy), amḷa (gooseberries) or fresh buttermilk with mint for relief. All these ingredients will bring down the pitta. Take another example. If due to aggravated or increased vāta doṣa you are not feeling hunger (that's due to low digestive fire), then you need to increase the amount of black pepper and ginger in your diet. Also, a mixture of ginger, lemon juice and a bit of Himalayan (saindha) salt helps relieve the gas and increase digestive fire. Similarly, carom seeds (ajwain) also help relieve the raised vāta due to indigestion. But if we continue to eat, say, tomatoes with chilli or sour yoghurt while having a pitta imbalance phase and chickpeas (chole) in vāta imbalance, we are sure to drive ourselves to sickness. And many chronic diseases will occur if we neglect this over and over again.

If we are aware of the food's qualities and our nature before we eat it, we can safely avoid an imbalance. This is how we design our food profile. For example, carom seeds are used to cook chickpeas as a preventive measure to keep vāta in check. Those whose vāta doṣa is vulnerable should either reduce chickpea in the diet or have more ginger and carom seeds. Similarly, fenugreek (methi) seeds can be used in sour preparations, such as sambar (south Indian sweet-sour lentil soup), kadhi (yoghurt curry with vegetables such as radish), idli or dosa batter, imli or raw mango preps with coconut. The bitterness in fenugreek seeds is pitta balancing.

Now, to understand your food profile, we're ready to discuss individual ingredients, their tridoṣa nature, rasa, guṇa and the corresponding impact on our tridoṣa nature. This section has very useful information; though you may find some of it a bit too much to take in at one go. Please feel free to skip a few ingredients and revisit them later, or read them as per your requirement. However, this information will help you design your diet profile, which concludes this section.

1. GRAINS (DHĀNYAM)

Ayurveda classifies grains under three categories;

A. Awned (grains with a covering to be removed, like rice and wheat),
B. Pods (like legumes/lentils, peas and beans), and
C. Grassy grains (millets)

A. Awned Grains (Śukam)

Rice: Rice is considered an excellent grain in Ayurveda because of its taste, ability to balance and nourish doṣas, build tissues and impart prāṇa or vitality. Some high-quality rice can even nourish and balance all three doṣas and be consumed by a person of any doṣa constitution and at any time (seasons or prescribed meals during the day). No wonder, rice is a staple food across the world. Moreover, it is gluten-free, has no allergic effects and is easy to digest.

Are the Carbohydrates in Rice Bad? There are many reports implying that carbohydrates, one of the main components of rice, are bad for health. But this is a blanket statement that is not true. Most animals that are herbivores eat a lot of carbohydrates and remain healthy. How so? Because animals mostly eat whole food. What we mostly eat is factory-processed refined/polished rice. There are two types of carbohydrates—one is complex and the other is simple. Both are found in rice as well as wheat.

Complex carbohydrates take longer to digest and simple ones are absorbed quickly. But complex carbohydrates are more beneficial because they digest slowly and supply energy in a sustained way. On the other hand, simple carbohydrates raise the blood sugar level quickly. Simple carbs provide an instant surge in the energy level to initiate actions. That means we should be ready to do some physical labour, or else the pancreas will be tasked to release more insulin to balance the sugar level in blood. Polished rice, bereft of complex carbohydrates, is a source of simple carbohydrates, and is not suitable, especially for people with diabetic problems. It is also not recommended for those who are at hereditary risk of diabetes.

Polished exposed grains are prone to attacks by pests. So, the standard practice to preserve polished rice, lentils, etc., is to fume these grains with pesticides. One of my friends, who is a senior scientist at India's top atomic research centre, told me that pesticides in exposed grains are more dangerous than pesticides in vegetables because vegetables have a skin to prevent the pesticide from entering the food. And ozonization can get rid of them to a fair extent. You can find devices producing ozone gas on the internet. But in case of polished grains, there is more pesticide exposure.

So, to conclude, the best rice is the organic variety, the one which is milled but not polished and stored without fumigation. Grains have both simple and complex carbs, but when we polish them, we lose the outer covering which contains complex carbs. This simple rule applies to all grains, awned or pods.

New Rice and Aged Rice: Rice needs to be aged for six to eight months before being processed, cooked and consumed. Freshly harvested rice can cause an imbalance in kapha, which may cause indigestion, bloating and cough. I remember how grains of rice used to be stored in villages of southern Odisha forty years ago. The farmers would dig large holes (10×10×15 feet) in front of their houses and then put straw in the holes to make a bed in the ditch. Then they would knit together straw to form a huge pouch. All the newly harvested awned grains of rice would be put in that pouch and sealed from all sides, to protect it from the rain and rats. Then it was covered with earth and mud, and a small dais over the hole would mark the location. They would call it a mine, because after seven to eight months, they would dig up the mud to extract the aged rice. The straw would keep the grains dry and warm. Upon ageing, the husk would come off easily as they would mill it manually. The rice thus obtained was wholesome. Aged rice cooks without clumping and manifests a sweet aroma. Most rice available now is not aged for long and packed and sold soon after harvesting.

However, freshly harvested rice cooked with milk is relished by many during festivals that follow the harvests.

Impact on Tridoṣa: Rice in general is sweet in taste, light to digest, alleviates or relieves pitta, may slightly imbalance kapha and vāta, strengthens the body, promotes growth, nourishes sattva guṇa and imparts satisfaction. There are hundreds of natural varieties of rice. Some grow in hot climates, some in the rainy season and yet some in winter. And of all those, raktasāli (sāli in Sanskrit means rice) is the best according to Ācārya Vāgabhaṭa. Rakta variety treats thirst and affliction of kapha, pitta and vāta doṣa. Another excellent variety of rice is called sasṭika which cures the impairment of all three doṣas, is tasty, stimulates digestive fire, promotes digestion, confers taste, is an aphrodisiac, nourishes the dhātus (tissues), is conducive to eat for people with diseases and mitigates fatigue, hunger and thirst. These two varieties of rice are still available commercially in India. Another very popular variety of rice is bāsmati. *Bās* means fragrance and *mati* means qualities or intelligence. Bāsmati means the rice with qualities of sweet fragrance. This variety is also known to treat afflictions of all the three doṣas. Whereas raktasāli mostly grows in the southern Indian climate, bāsmati grows only once a year in the Indo-Gangetic Plain beneath the Himalayan sub-ranges (Dehradun) of northern India. Twenty years ago, whenever I would cook bāsmati, the fragrance would spread all over the house. Unfortunately, the quality of this bāsmati rice has deteriorated drastically in the last two decades, probably due to genetic modification, cultivation in unfavourable climates and growing commercial demand.

Rice and Millet: As rice is easy to digest and wholesome, it is considered better than other grains. Rice is known to impart a lot of sattva guṇa and is considered particularly good for those who are engaged in intellectual activity throughout the day. Since they are not engaged in hard labour, they need food that is easy to digest. On the other hand, millets are advised when muscular prowess (rajo guṇa or passion) needs to be used. Millets are easily digested too, but need to be soaked in water for seven to eight hours. Millets impart a lot of physical strength, strengthen bones and joints.

Recently, a lot has been said about the benefits of millets over rice as millet is cultivated from grass, which grows easily and requires less water, and fewer chemical fertilizers and pesticides than rice. Rice requires a lot of care, from the time the saplings are sowed, to growing, harvesting, storing, processing and cooking. But when done properly, it imparts the best of health.

Millets, on the other hand, grow easily and do not require much care for processing and storing. Millets are mostly spared from chemicals and organic varieties are more easily available than rice. So, it is safer to consume millets, but it's not ideal for those who are engaged in heavy intellectual activities.

Wheat: Known as *goḍhūma*, wheat is also considered an excellent grain in Ayurveda. Whereas rice is light to digest, wheat is heavy and generally requires higher digestive fire. So, people like to eat wheat in winter, when the digestive fire is high. People in central and northern India prefer to eat rotis (flat fresh bread) while people in the southern parts of the country prefer rice throughout the year, as the winter is mild in these regions. In some regions, people prefer to eat rotis in the evening when the weather is cooler.

In general, wheat reverses the afflictions of vāta and pitta, imparts firmness and strength to the body, and promotes repair. It is heavy in potency, cool to digest and sweet in taste. According to Vāgabhaṭa, the small variety of wheat, which grows in central provinces (Madhya Pradesh), is considered the best, because although wheat in general is heavy to digest, this variety, known by the name Nāndimukhi, is light. Another small variety, known as Madhuli, still grows in Madhya Pradesh and is considered to be of very high quality.

Similar to polished rice, white flour is also considered not good as it is not wholesome. Traditionally, plain flour would be produced by stone-grinding the wheat and then sifting the flour to remove the bran (husk) and germ (hard seed inside the wheat grain). The removed husk is best for animal feed. With time (nearly four to six weeks), the flour in contact with air turns white. This process of obtaining white flour is called ageing. Then the flour is kneaded for a long time (for half hour or more) to activate the gluten and make bread, confectionary (baklava, khaja, cakes, etc.), savouries (samosa, etc.) and pizzas. The word pav-roti for bread is named so in India because earlier people used to knead the dough with their feet in commercial bakeries. Feet in Hindi are called pav.

The bran and germ have a lot of minerals, such as iron, zinc, calcium and potassium along with proteins, enzymes, vitamins and healthy fatty acids. The endosperm, or the white flour of wheat, is mostly starch with some protein and carbohydrates. So naturally it is not as healthy as whole wheat flour. For obtaining whole wheat flour, the grinding is done until the husk and germ turn to powder as well. However, it still needs to be sifted afterwards. But modern rolling steel mills remove the bran and germ completely. And on top of that they add chemicals like benzoyl peroxide or fume it with chlorine to bleach the flour quickly.

Bleaching agents like chlorine gas also alter the structure of proteins in the flour through oxidation. This further helps to improve the softness of baked goods. But the problem with chemically bleached flour is that the residual levels of both benzoyl peroxide and its reaction product benzoic acid can cause health issues. Some researchers point to benzoyl peroxide as a cause of tumors (though not carcinogen). As such, benzoyl peroxide, which is an explosive, disqualifies bleached flours as organic. Most commercially produced breads, biscuits, cakes, cookies and baked products contain chemically bleached white flour and should thus be avoided. If you want to use white flour for cooking, try to buy unbleached white flour. It will be more expensive as the process is not as popular today.

Barley: This grain is mentioned in the Vedas and used for auspicious sacrifices. It is astringent and sweet in taste and vitiates impairment caused by kapha and pitta, but increases vāta (due to its astringent taste). This is recommended to be eaten when one has a fever, as it is cold yet treats pitta and kapha imbalances.

B. Beans/Grains from Pods

These consist mostly of legumes and beans. These protein pods are heavier to digest than awned grains. They normally aggravate or increase vāta doṣa. An imbalance of vāta causes constipation, similar to how air trapped in a water pipe hinders the flow of water.

Moong dal or moong beans are the lightest among all legumes and easy to digest. However, they do not impart much strength. The black variety of moong (which is a rare breed) is known to mitigate the imbalances of all the three doṣas, especially vāta, whereas the green variety relieves kapha and pitta. That means the black variety can be eaten any time, whereas the green variety needs to be avoided if vāta doṣa is too high. For others, it can still be consumed anytime as it is easy to digest. Even those with low digestive fire can absorb the proteins in the legumes. Green moong also provides nourishment for the eyes.

The next best variety is pigeon pea legume or toor/harar dal. This pacifies kapha and pitta, but slightly aggravates vāta. It is also very popular for its taste and nourishment. The vāta can be balanced by adding spices such as asafoetida (hing) and ginger. Similarly, if cooked with ghee, this legume balances all the three doṣas and becomes light to digest too. But those with vāta imbalance are advised to avoid it, especially when the digestive fire is weak. Some categorize this dal as rājasic, but I have found extensive use of this legume in all the Vishnu temples of India and believe it has a sāttvic impact on the mind. Vishnu is the Lord of sattva guṇa, and thus we categorize this dal under sattva guṇa.

Other examples of beans are Bengal gram (chana dal), red kidney beans (rajma), chickpea and black gram (urad dal). The order of heaviness to digest increases from Bengal gram to black gram. They raise vāta and also pitta, the latter as they are hot in potency. The excess pitta affects the blood (temperature) and the skin. Black gram, rajma and chole are very heavy and should be consumed in winter. In south India, where the chill of winter is absent, black gram is ground with a high proportion of rice and water, and then fermented to make it light for consumption. These heavy legumes impart a lot of strength and should be consumed by those who are healthy and physically active through the day, for example, those engaged in military disciplines. Black gram has more protein than many kinds of meat, and a vegetarian can get all the protein they require from these grains.

C. Grassy Grains or Millets

Sorghum/Great Millet, known as jawār in India, is used to make gluten-free rotis or bhākri, which is also a flat bread. This flour is good for those with gluten intolerance and weak digestion, or both. Gluten intolerance is mostly due to the lack of one's ability to digest glutenous protein. White flour has 12–14 per cent gluten, which lends a certain kind of taste, consistency and sponginess to bread and cakes and provides strength for the expanded structure to hold shape as these bake.

Sorghum relieves kapha and pitta and increases vāta, though according to Vāgabhaṭa the white variety of sorghum is light to digest and treats vitiation of all three doṣas. Sorghum is sweet in taste, imparts strength, and treats haemorrhoids. Jawāri/sorghum in general is easy to digest and provides a lot of strength. When the weather turns hot and arid, the digestive fire naturally slows down. This grain is recommended to be eaten in such weather for strength. On the other hand, wheat in such weather may impair pitta doṣa as it is more difficult to digest. This results in ailments of the digestive tract. Therefore, people in south India hardly consume wheat as the climate there is hot throughout the year.

Pearl millet or bājrā is, recommended to be eaten in winter as it is hot in potency. Five times richer in iron than sorghum, this millet is a good gluten-free substitute for wheat in winter. Bājrā neutralizes pitta and vāta. But because it is hot in nature, it neutralizes kapha too. Both jawāri and bājrā are served with molten ghee. Ghee neutralizes the dryness of jawāri which otherwise disturbs vāta, and cools down the hot potency of bājrā.

Another great millet is Finger Millet, popularly known as rāgi (also as nāchni, māndua) and is easy to digest while supplying a good deal of protein and minerals like calcium. It increases vāta but does not disturb pitta and kapha much. So, it is easy to digest but requires some ghee or oil to balance the vāta. Also, this extra vāta can be utilized through heavy physical activities. Compared with wheat and other millets, the protein content is low, but that's also why it is easier to digest and assimilate. It is enriched with more calcium than other grains and is very useful to strengthen our bones and teeth. It also has a high iron content. This is consumed all over India throughout the year.

Here I would like take a detour and discuss amaranth. Amaranth is an excellent class of whole seeds. This Indian superfood, which is locally known by the name Rām Dānā or Rajgirā, is not a millet because the leaves and stems are used as vegetables and the plant falls in the botanical family of spinach. However, the characteristics of amaranth seeds resemble millets, and it's prepared in a similar way too. Technically, it is not a grain and therefore it is recommended to be eaten on Ekādaśi (eleventh lunar days) and other grain-fasting days. This food is a storehouse of minerals and vitamins. Amaranth is similar to finger millet in its impact on tridoṣa and also rich in calcium and iron.

2. VEGETABLES

Ayurveda classifies vegetables under six categories:

A. Leaf or Patra Śāka
B. Flower or Puṣpa Śāka
C. Vegetable or Phala Śāka
D. Stem or Nāḷa or Danḍa Śāka
E. Tuber and Root or Kanda and Muḷa Śāka
F. Mushroom or Samsvedaja (born of own heat or sweat)

The order of digestive power required to digest a vegetable increases from leafy vegetables to root. According to Ayurvedic principles, all types of vegetables can cause constipation (as they aggravate vāta), are heavy, dry, produce excess faecal matter and flatus. Vegetables are also thought to weaken bones, destroy vision, complexion, blood, semen and intellect, cause greying of hair and deteriorate memory. In other words, all edible vegetables are ever ready to destroy the body! This is described so in an Ayurvedic dietary treatise called *Bhojanakutuhalam*. But what does this mean, and why do we eat vegetables then? All this is true only if the vegetables are consumed raw. Raw vegetables require a lot of digestive fire for the simple reason that plants and animals are different living systems and thus are incompatible with the human body. As a result, excess amḷa or sour taste is generated during digestion, which impacts the body negatively. Therefore, to balance this, one must prepare and cook the vegetables appropriately to make them digestible and useful for the body and mind. Vegetables must be cooked with oil or ghee. Even boiled vegetables need to be topped with some oil or ghee.

But then how do herbivores like elephants consume nearly 250 kg (500 pounds) of raw leaves and vegetables every single day? It is possible for them to do so as they have much longer intestines than humans.

Humans are omnivores, so our intestines are not as long as herbivores and not as short as carnivores. Carnivores have short intestines as the raw meat tends to decompose quickly. With our intermediate length of intestine, we need to consume cooked food, whether vegetables or meat. Some people argue that raw food has maximum prāṇa or life-energy, and by cooking we lose some prāṇa. While it's true, we wouldn't be able to digest and thus assimilate the excess prāṇa in vegetables anyway. The body cannot absorb all the prāṇa as digestion is never 100 per cent and some prāṇa is lost through faecal excreta. The nutrients thus lost become food for other animals. However, some vegetables, which are easier to digest, such as cucumber, can be eaten raw. Or in the cold, when the digestive fire is high, we may consume certain raw vegetables, such as carrots.

Ayurveda describes vegetables as saḍras pūrṇa, meaning full and complete, with six tastes that are essential for a complete meal. We will discuss all six types of vegetables with a few examples and their impact on tridoṣa.

A. Leaf or Patra Śāka

Among all edible vegetables, leaves are the easiest to digest. Which is why they form a majority of ingredients in salads. However, it is still important to prepare a salad the right way to make sure it is easily digested. Adding black pepper boosts the digestive fire, while lemon aids in digestion. Oil ignites the digestive fire and also balances vāta (which causes dryness as well as bloating and flatus). So, it is best to use salad dressing. Blend together about half a teaspoon of black pepper powder, quarter teaspoon salt, two tablespoons of extra virgin olive oil, one teaspoon of fresh lemon juice and four tablespoons of water. Use this with fresh salad leaves and salad raw vegetables like cucumber, tender carrots and tender radish. Another dressing I personally like is a combination of pure organic coconut oil, salt, fresh lemon juice and green chilli mashed manually in a stone mortar with a pestle. There are many other recipes of salad dressing complying with Ayurvedic principles that can be adapted depending upon one's doṣa constitution. You can find more in the recipes section. Fresh raw leaves should ideally be eaten during winters, when the digestive fire is high, and bugs and pests are absent. In the West, people eat a lot of salads in the summer, but as the temperature ranges between 10 and 25° Celsius, it is similar to winter in India.

Eating raw salad leaves, especially the ones that grow close to the earth, in summer in India is not recommended as the leaves may carry bugs or invisible eggs. These can leak into the blood and cause severe health problems. However, salads prepared using fresh cucumber and similar vegetables, which grow on creepers and have a thick protective skin, are prescribed and safe to consume.

Leafy Vegetables: Cooking leaves over a fire helps mitigate the problems we have discussed above. But it is important to first beat the leaves together a few times to get rid of bugs and eggs before washing and chopping.

Generally, a good way to cook leafy vegetables is to first sauté asafoetida in ghee/oil with crushed black pepper in a pan. The washed and chopped leafy vegetables are then added to this to be stir-fried. Salt and turmeric are added, and the greens stir-fried till the leaves are well cooked, there is no water left in the pan and the oil resurfaces a bit. This can be served with a slice of fresh lemon or buttermilk on the side. To preserve the freshness, always cook leafy vegetables in open pots without a lid. Sometimes, I cook leafy vegetables with a combination of compatible vegetables, such as sweet potatoes (helps to absorb the excess water of leaves) and pumpkins, both diced small. Some use a few teaspoons of yellow moong beans to add flavour and also absorb the excess water. Using freshly grated coconut to dress the cooked leafy vegetables also enhances the taste. As always, it is important to be careful while adding a new ingredient and understand how the combination will interact with the doṣas of the person eating the food. I would add a bit of grated ginger while combining sweet potatoes with leafy vegetables to check the excess accompanying vāta.

In the category of leafy vegetables one must look beyond spinach. I have seen a wide variety, up to fifty-eight, being sold in the farmer's market of Navadwip, a small town in West Bengal.

The best of all leafy vegetables, according to Ayurvedic authorities, is vathuā, known in English as Chenopodium album or lamb's quarter. This delightedly tasteful leafy vegetable not only mitigates all the three doṣas but is also effective in checking internal haemorrhage, eliminating worms, strengthening the body and evacuating excreta.

The leaves of the amaranth or rajgirā plants are also extremely nutritious and are known to kindle impaired gastric fire. These should be cooked in sesame oil with asafoetida and salt. It treats the damage caused by excess kapha and pitta doṣas in people of all prakṛti types.

Another variety that should be included in the diet is fresh methikā or fenugreek leaves. Although slightly bitter in taste, this leafy vegetable adds a beautiful fragrance to the kitchen and whets the appetite. The chopped leaves should first be boiled with salt and turmeric with little or no water. Then the excess water should be squeezed out and the tender cooked pulpy leaves sautéed in ghee and asafoetida. Methikā is good for treating imbalanced kapha and thus alleviates bronchitis and respiratory system issues.

The caṇā or leaves of Bengal gram/chickpea plants are also nutritious and prepared by washing the chopped caṇā and sautéing with ghee, asafoetida, salt and turmeric. Once it is 80–90 per cent cooked through, one should add freshly made rice powder (just enough to bind the vegetables to form a single mass) with ginger and cook till the moisture dries out and the ghee starts to separate. Continue to cook in this separated ghee to bring out the taste. This leafy vegetable causes a good deal of imbalance in kapha and vāta, so ginger (known for balancing vāta) and ghee (known for balancing both vāta and pitta) should be used liberally. People whose vāta doṣa is vulnerable and increases upon even a slight change in diet having vāta prominence need to have more ginger.

The way this vegetable is prepared is heavy, and it takes time to digest. However, it is very good for cardiac health. Spinach too is heavy to digest and requires a bit more ginger and ghee. It increases kapha and vāta, but treats pitta-related ailments. Despite being a green leafy vegetable, spinach is known to cause ophthalmic ailments.

On the other hand, fragrant dill leaves (satapuṣpā) alleviate ophthalmic diseases while mitigating kapha and vāta doṣas. Similarly, poyica (*poi sāk*) relieves vāta and pitta, is cool in potency (so it can be prepared with mustard paste which is heating), nourishes the entire body and induces sleep (so it induces tamas and people strictly desiring sattva avoid eating poyica). Moringa (leaves from drumstick plants) is yet another leafy vegetable that is unprecedented in its taste, flavour and fragrance. It is cooked with yellow moong beans and freshly grated coconut. Moringa is a very rich source of iron.

I personally cook around two cups of thick blanched and puréed spinach with two tablespoons of ginger paste, a quarter cup of chopped tomatoes and half a teaspoon of Himalayan pink salt in three tablespoons of ghee. Ginger and tomatoes are cooked in heated ghee over medium to low fire for about fifteen minutes or so with salt before adding the spinach purée. Then the whole combination is cooked for about five minutes. Do not cover the dish while cooking to maintain the green colour. Serve immediately with hot rotis topped with ghee. I cook mustard greens (sarson ka sāg) in the same way except the mustard leaves, instead of blanching, are boiled for twenty-five to thirty minutes over a medium fire before being drained and puréed.

Try this simple recipe. I am sure you will like it. Tomatoes are not used very often in Ayurvedic methods of cooking as they are thought to impair all the three doṣas. But ginger and ghee are likely to take care of that. If you wish, you may remove the tomatoes and serve a slice of lemon and buttermilk alongside the roti and sarson ka sāg.

B. Flower or Puṣpa Śāka

Many varieties of flowers are cooked for health benefits. We will discuss a few. Agastya, popularly known as agati (in Tāmil) or shevari (in Marāthi) is very healthy and highly recommended. The agati tree's tender leaves, green fruit, and flowers can be eaten by themselves as a vegetable or mixed into curries or salads. Flowers may be dipped in chickpea flour batter and fried in ghee. Another way to prepare these flowers is to boil them in buttermilk along with the tender fruits. After that, it is fried in ghee with asafoetida and other spices, such as cumin, coriander powder, turmeric and salt. This preparation mitigates kapha and pitta doṣas, and has a cooling effect that helps to relieve recurring fever. Agati flowers are harvested and cooked in many parts of south-east Asia. The tree grows abundantly without needing much attention and blooms with many flowers. I would often pluck and cook this flower in Govardhan Eco Village situated near Mumbai.

The agati tree has a lot of medicinal properties and every part of it—roots, bark, fruit, leaf and gum—can be used to make Ayurvedic medicines. Because agati trees grow quickly, they used to be a major source of firewood for cooking. Now, these trees are grown to make paper.

Banana flowers are very popular in central, eastern, western and southern India, and are considered a delicacy. After removing the stalk, the flowers are chopped and washed and then boiled in water with salt and turmeric. After it has cooked well, the excess water is removed and the cooked vegetable is stir-fried in ghee with asafoetida, pepper and other appropriate spices. It could be commonly used cumin seeds and turmeric or spices according to a person's tridoṣa. For example, we can add a little ginger paste to alleviate impaired vāta doṣa. This neutralizes kapha, pitta and vāta doṣa ailments and is suitable for people of all doṣas. The pitta doṣa is especially addressed as a result of the astringent taste of banana flowers. It prevents bloating.

Araṇi is known as arni in Hindi and Agnimantha in Sanskrit. As the name suggests, the woods of dry arni are used to ignite fire for auspicious yajñas. Naturally, this food is hot in potency. Therefore, for best results, this flower is stored in clean water for seven nights and then boiled in buttermilk. Afterwards, it is stir-fried with ghee and asafoetida, salt and pepper. This preparation balances all the three doṣas (tridoṣa samanah), strengthens heart function, and checks flatulence and bloating. The flower is anti-inflammatory, relieves ophthalmic ailments and eliminates poisonous or toxic effects.

A discussion about edible flowers is incomplete without nim. Nim flowers in the budding stage have tender leaves that are first washed well and then roasted with ghee and salt. These should be cooked till the buds turn brownish. This preparation is consumed while warm and as a starter. My mother would mix rice flour and asafoetida to make a thick batter. She would then coat the buds in it and pan fry them as patties. This simple preparation, although bitter, is irresistible. It stimulates gastric fire and prevents a lot of diseases. Usually, the flowers appear on nim plants towards the end of the summer season. Consuming the flowers a few times can protect the body from infectious diseases that spread in the rainy season. It also relieves ailments manifested by imbalance of kapha and pitta doṣa, cures all kind of skin diseases, ulcers, and is good to have if you suffer from diabetes and urinary diseases. Some prepare this item with tiny pieces of eggplant to moderate the bitterness.

The last flower I would like to discuss is pumpkin flower. Especially because pumpkin trees grow practically in all seasons and climates across the world. Although, as a vegetable, pumpkin disturbs the balance of all the tridoṣa, the flower is very useful. It balances vāta and helps strengthen bones. It is also pitta pacifying as it's cold in potency. It nourishes kapha and thus the immune system too. One way of preparing it is to steam the flowers and eat them with a sprinkle of pure cold pressed mustard oil or cold pressed extra virgin olive oil, and salt and pepper. Or it can be pan fried with asafoetida and pepper. But my favourite way of eating it is to pan fry it in a batter of rice flour and spices such as turmeric, cumin powder and asafoetida.

C. Vegetable or Phala Śāka

Non-leafy vegetables require careful cooking as these are tougher to digest. Among all vegetables, the ones that grow on creepers are better for health than the rest. They are easier and lighter to digest, contain more minerals and vitamins and less starch or carbohydrates. For example, various types of gourds (bottle gourd or lauki, paṭola or pointed gourd, bitter gourd or karela, ridged gourd or turi (in Hindi) or round gourd or white pumpkin, etc.) and squash (red pumpkin or kaddu, zucchini, etc.). Ayurveda recommends preparation of these vegetables for nourishing health more than root vegetables. I have observed that vegetables that are easier to digest float in water when they are chopped into pieces, while those that are difficult to digest sink to the bottom of the pot. Floating indicates that these are not dense and will be digested more easily in the stomach.

Generally, vegetables from creepers float on water. All these vegetables have their own intrinsic qualities (guṇa) and cooking them a certain way brings out their best qualities. One vegetable that is wholesome, truly healthy and mentioned in all Ayurvedic texts is kuṣmāṇḍa or ash gourd. It is available in two varieties; tender and matured. The matured variety is very tasty, with a sweet flavour, slightly alkaline, mitigates all three doṣas, augments digestive fire, is easily digestible, cures mental disorders, and cleanses the urinary bladder. A mature ash gourd should be chopped, washed and cooked in ghee with asafoetida and black pepper. Then it should be cooked further with thin fresh buttermilk, salt, turmeric and roasted cumin powder till it is done. Adding curry leaves makes it tastier.

Another vegetable that is sought out for its taste and is a great appetizer (helps to defeat aruchi or aversion to eating) is brinjal or eggplant. Small green tender eggplants, when cut in two and fried with ghee and spiced with sautéed asafoetida, black pepper and salt are good for stimulating hunger. Besides stimulating the taste buds, eggplant helps ignite gastric fire, mitigates vāta, supports the heart's functions, promotes semen production and is easily digested.

Bitter gourd cooked in ghee and cumin seeds purifies the blood, regulates the blood sugar level, improves skin health, treats kapha and pitta doṣas, but increases vāta doṣa. So, it is best to cook it in more oil or ghee. But eat in moderation so that you do not consume too much ghee or oil. One more recipe is included in Section Five (Yogi Plate).

D. Stem/Stalk Vegetables or Naḷa or Daṇḍa Sāka

There are very few varieties of this category of vegetable. We will discuss two types. One is banana stems, which is available in warm humid climates, such as areas from central to southern India. Banana stems are removed from a mature banana tree. The soft tender core is used for cooking. After removing the excess fibre, the stem is diced into small cubes and boiled in buttermilk with a little turmeric and salt for eight to ten minutes. After draining the liquid, the stem is sautéed in ghee, chopped fresh ginger and drizzled with fresh chopped coriander/cilantro leaves. This preparation is very cooling for the stomach and repairs the damage in the intestines. It also helps in menorrhagia (or vaginal bleeding), stimulates the taste buds, kindles gastric fire and balances pitta and vāta doṣa. It is very useful to keep the stomach light and cool.

Tender mustard stems with soft foliage (sarson ka sāg) are example of a stem vegetable. This is more popular in northern India and eaten in the winter. The clean, washed stalks are chopped and boiled in water or thin buttermilk. The pulp is then fried in a good quantity of ghee, asafoetida and black pepper. Finally, rock salt is added for taste. The ghee helps neutralize the excess vāta (and thus dryness) of the stalk vegetable. As such, winter brings a lot of dryness, and vāta tends to be high at such a time. So, one need not be annoyed by the presence of floating ghee in this preparation unless one suffers from obesity or chronic heart ailments. This preparation mitigates the problem of kapha and vāta, the two problems associated with winter. It also helps to heal wounds, itching, alleviates obstinate skin problems and stimulates the taste buds. Again, skin problems are concurrent with winter.

In the West, the two most prominent stems used are asparagus and celery stems. Whereas asparagus is mostly consumed whole, celery stems with tender leaves make delicious aromatic soups and chutneys. Celery has the ability to balance kapha and vāta and is good for relieving abdominal pain. It is hot in potency and thus good for consuming in winter. Asparagus increases vāta but balances kapha. It's useful in purifying blood and is considered an excellent diuretic. It should be avoided if vāta doṣa is imbalanced, as it causes excess dryness.

In south-east Asia, lemon grass stalks are also used a lot in soups and curries, and add to the fragrance and flavour of Thai curries in particular. It balances vāta and kapha, helps raise the gastric fire and can treat coughs and colds. I prepare lemongrass tea using both stalks and leaves, along with some grated ginger, a few drops of lemon juice and khadi sakar (rock sugar candy). This tea helps to rejuvenate the senses and mind.

E. Tubers and Roots or Kanda and Muḷa Sāka

Tubers and roots are the toughest vegetables to digest, as they are more dense and heavy. Especially in places that have a cold climate, the warmth of the soil incubates tubers and roots as the upper part of the plants cannot fructify much. These vegetables are generally known to increase vāta more than any other. Nature encourages the growth of such vegetables in winter so that the extra vāta shakes people out of lethargy, and lends energy. In winter, one is blessed with extra digestive fire, (pitta is activated more to fight the chill outside the body) which helps digest such vegetables. However, some exceptional tubers can be consumed throughout the year if cooked the right way. We will discuss a few here.

Suraṇa or elephant yam, though a tuber, is light to digest yet effective in treating diseases caused by imbalanced kapha, such as cough and bronchitis. This also soothes ailments caused by imbalanced pitta, such as piles. Oil your palms while washing and peeling the yam, as it may make your palms itch. The vegetable may either be diced or cut into two-inch long rectangular (finger shape) pieces. It should then be boiled with something sour, such as tamarind leaves or thin, sour buttermilk. This helps make sure that the yam does not cause an itchy sensation in the throat. Once boiled, the diced vegetables should be cooked with sesame oil, asafoetida, pepper, turmeric, curry leaves and salt. The pieces can be deep fried in mustard oil till they turn brown and crispy. After draining the oil, toss the pieces with powdered spices, such as dry mango powder, black pepper powder, roasted cumin powder and dry ginger powder. I would cook yam this way when living in the ashram, and it was extremely popular among the residents. These fries are a good alternative to French fries. However, the fried yam's beneficial and medicinal properties are less potent than those of boiled yam. Suraṇa is also baked by peeling the skin and then mashing it with mustard oil, salt, black pepper, lemon juice and ginger. This is called bhartā.

Other vegetables can also be used to prepare bhartā, especially eggplant. It is better to roast it over a wood fire rather than an electric oven, as the wood fire steadily roasts vegetables while simultaneously maintaining the moisture in the vegetable. When the wood burns, carbon dioxide and water are produced naturally. This moisture retains the rasa/juicy taste of the vegetables whereas an electric oven may dry up the vegetables and increase vāta doṣa as one of the impact of the vāta doṣa is dryness. Cooking over gas is also not as good as cooking over a wood fire, but better than an electric oven as the gas fire produces some moisture while burning.

Because roots such as potatoes and sweet potatoes potentially disturb vāta doṣa, it is general Ayurvedic advice that they should be prepared with a good quantity of ginger and sharp pungent (kaṭu) oil, such as mustard, as both of these ingredients are antidotes for vāta doṣa. Ghee can be added on the top if pitta doṣa is too prominent. These vegetables should be consumed in winter or a cold climate and should be avoided if vāta doṣa is already high.

F. Mushroom or Samsvedaja (Born of Own Heat or Sweat)

Mushrooms mostly grow in dark and damp surroundings, such as paddy straw that has not been dried properly. This is why mushrooms are considered tāmasic. Ayurveda advises not to consume mushrooms as these are known to be doṣāla or one that aggravates and disturbs all the three doṣas. So, most practising yogis and people cooking according to sāttvic methods do not eat mushrooms.

3. DAIRY (KṢIRAṀ)

In the Vedas, seven personalities are honoured as mothers: mātā or one's own mother, rāja mātā or queen, guru mātā or wife of spiritual master, dhātṛi or nurse/midwife, bhudevi or mother earth and gau mātā or cow. Mother is a symbol of selfless service rendered with gratitude.

In the 1960s, when the government of the state of Odisha decided to build residential quarters for its employees, it included a cowshed in every house. As a child, I lived in one of these houses for many years. We had multiple cows in the shed. Each of them had a name. And every time a calf was born, our home would have an overwhelming supply of milk. Of course, this was after the calf had got enough to drink. Sometimes the calf would sneak out from its allotted space and drink milk from its mother unchecked, and as a result, fall sick, without exception. This is because a cow produces far more milk than the little calf's stomach can handle. Centuries ago, it was considered that the milk was for the entire family. She provided for all the members and was regarded as a mother figure. Cows were kept as though they were a part of the family and were never meant for sale. They were only gifted. A society where the land, animals and people are respected will be blessed with a happiness that permeates every corner and prevails in everyone's heart.

The milk from the cows in our house was divine and the taste is ingrained in my mind. Twenty-five years later, when I was living in Mumbai, one of my friends in the ashram got some pure milk all the way from Rajasthan. As the head cook, I was asked to verify the milk's quality. When I sipped that milk, my memories resurfaced, and my smile confirmed everything.

Some nutritionists now believe that humans shouldn't consume animal milk. They are correct to say this about the milk that is mass produced, which comes from cows who are kept like machines for milk and meat. They are fed artificially designed food and injected with hormones to draw more milk. The milk is processed to skim the fat, and sometimes other things are added to enhance certain qualities. Thus, the pure natural form and the tridoṣa prakṛti of the milk is disturbed. So, it is unfit for consumption from an Ayurvedic perspective too. According to Ayurveda, milk which is not boiled within two to three hours of milking, causes disorder and thus is not fit for consumption. On the other hand, Ayurveda proclaims that fresh and pure cow milk is the most suitable diet that nature can offer. It is more compatible with human bodies than grains or vegetables. This is because we drink the mother's milk as infants. And later, we slowly include grains, vegetables and fruits in our diet, which are basically from the plant kingdom or different life-systems. In other words, milk and meat are more easily processed by the human body than vegetables as the human body itself is made up of milk and flesh.

But meat is a product of violence (tāmasic) and so needs to be avoided, if not completely then as much as possible, whereas milk is a product of goodness (sāttvic). One can survive on just pure cow milk. Many wandering saints regard cow milk as the best form of non-violent food that can be consumed fresh without processing. Apart from cows, Ayurveda speaks about other animals that give milk too.

To derive the best benefits, the milk should be fresh and from cows who are well cared for. Secondly, the cow's fodder should be sourced from nature and be completely organic. In general, *Bhojanakutuhalam* states that milk instantly increases semen production, imparts intelligence, wisdom and retentive power (memory), promotes growth and is enlivening, strengthening and conducive for all beings. Milk prevents ageing, increases life expectancy and rejoins broken tissues (including bones). It is also known to increase ojas. Milk is described as a rasāyana in the Ayurveda, which means it is capable of curing many ailments. Milk aggravates kapha but balances pitta and vāta. In Ayurvedic texts, milk has been described in five different forms. These are milk, yoghurt, butter, cheese and ghee (clarified butter).

It is best to boil milk by adding an equal quantity of water and then reducing it to the original amount. Boiling it for a long time makes the milk lighter to digest, apart from neutralizing all the pathogens. Milk can be consumed in the morning, afternoon and evening, but should be avoided at night as it requires some physical activity to be digested. However, it is important that we consume fresh, organic cow milk. Those with increased kapha doṣa should ideally drink milk with cardamom, dry ginger and saffron. Milk stored in copper, gold and silver pots alleviates vāta, pitta and kapha respectively. Milk boiled in an iron pot balances pitta and kapha, and kills worm-infestations in the intestine. Milk boiled in *kansa* (a traditional Indian metal alloy made up of 78 per cent copper and 22 per cent tin) balances all three doṣas and is considered a rasāyana. It is a good idea to look for kansa and silver pots to cook with it. These are still available in markets in India.

Yoghurt, curd or dahi is obtained by fermenting milk with the help of a bacterial culture. At a certain temperature (35–45° Celsius) the bacteria multiplies quickly and curdles milk to become dahi within six–eight hours. At the beginning, when the curd is thin, it disturbs or impairs all the three doṣas, but when it thickens (after six to eight hours), the curd is svādu or tasteful. Svādu curd increases kapha and pitta, but balances vāta. After six to eight hours, curd turns sour, and is called sour curd, which impairs kapha and pitta doṣas aggressively. But curd in general increases gastric fire as it is hot in potency. Salt with curd reduces the impact on kapha, while sugar increases it. Therefore lassi (sugar and yoghurt smoothies) and srikhand (another sweet preparation from yoghurt) contain dry ginger powder (sunthi), cardamom (elāichi) and saffron (kesar), which check the imbalance it can cause in kapha prakṛti.

Traditionally, curd is prepared in clay pots. Unlike metallic pots, clay pots are porous and also known as breathing pots. They naturally keep yoghurt and buttermilk cool and prevent fermentation/souring naturally. Usually they would keep it in such pots throughout the day and keep serving from that. In the night, a fresh lot would be kept for fermentation to be consumed for the following day. But now, when we have refrigeration easily available, we can store vegetables in the fridge for a week or less and similarly store yoghurt too. Make sure you cover it with a tight lid.

However, making it fresh every night, which takes only eight to ten minutes, and consuming it the following day would be the best practice. Buy some unglazed clay pots, wash them and soak them in water for a night before using for setting yoghurt. Change the clay pot every week or so. In cold weather this may not work. Use an insulated pot to set yoghurt with slight access to atmospheric air in cold weather. Never set yoghurt in copper, aluminium or kansa pots, as the metals will leach into the yoghurt.

Living in a nuclear family with mounting responsibilities, simple tasks like these can seem difficult and time-consuming. Also, in a metropolis, one rarely has access to fresh milk. Considering all these factors, we can refrigerate food ingredients as per our requirement. But as much as possible, try to eat fresh food and adhere to the traditional way of cooking.

Cheese is generally made by fermenting milk. Caraka-Saṃhitā mentions takrapinḍa, which is obtained by separating the water/whey from yoghurt using a piece of thin cloth. Takrapinḍa, which can be classified as cheese, is used to make srikhand. Yoghurt is made by fermenting milk using lactobacillus bacteria, a living organism that thrives on the lactose in milk. This bacteria releases an enzyme called lactase, which acts on the lactose and converts it into lactic acid, which in turn causes the milk to curdle by acting on milk proteins. Bacteria keep multiplying as the milk curdles. Besides curdling the milk, the bacteria are helpful in maintaining the flora of our gut. Just like fish and other organisms keep a pond clean, these bacteria keep our gut clean. Research has shown how this bacteria helps remove the bad bacteria and stop diarrhoea. It also facilitates, under certain conditions, production of good cholesterol. Antibiotic pills kill both the bad as well as the good bacteria in our gut. The bacteria in fermented food is what helps replenish it.

In the western world, cheese is also made by fermenting milk with enzymes obtained from the stomach of an unweaned (tender) mammal, known as rennet. Some people believe that cheese was formed when some desert travellers transported milk in a bag made from a camel's stomach, which caused it to curdle and become cheese.

Everyone's stomach has enzymes that act on milk. But rennet in a tender mammal's (such as goat, lamb and calf) stomach acts gently so that the food is absorbed well and nourishes the tender calf's body. Grown-up mammals, who subsist on vegetables, have low or no rennet.

How many calves had to be killed for cheese-making is unthinkable. In the early 1990s, because of the high demand for cheese, the irregular supply of calf rennet and the consequently fluctuating prices of cheese, genetic engineers devised ways to artificially manufacture rennet. They copied the gene of the rennet enzyme and engineered it into living microorganisms to produce enzymes like rennet. So, rennet was then commercially produced through genetically controlled microbial cultures so that it can be used to ferment milk and make cheese. Now the process has evolved further, and most of these enzymes are produced using a simpler fermentation technique called Fermentation-Produced Chymosin (FPC). According to the Wisconsin Center for Dairy Research, USA, only 5 per cent of cheese is made from calf rennet and the remaining produced from these genetically replicated cultures. However, the cheese thus obtained is not considered a genetically modified organism (GMO) as the rennet produced by genetically modified microbes is pure and the cheese is considered vegetarian. Ayurvedic texts do not touch upon this, as all these are modern procedures, but it does speak of processes similar to those of fermenting milk to make yoghurt.

Another way of making fresh cheese is to curdle hot milk with a sharp acid, such as citric acid from lemons. This fresh cheese is called paneer or cottage cheese. Fresh mozzarella is a similar product. These types of fresh cheese can be classified as sāttvic. But aged cheese which is stored for a long time is not sāttvic. The practice of storing and ageing cheese exists because there are places on the planet where nothing grows in the winter and fresh food is tough to come by. Thus, cheese was a useful means of subsistence during such times.

Takrapinḍa, paneer or cheese promotes development of tissues, enhances strength, is an aphrodisiac and is heavy for digestion. As it is heavy, it is not as popular in hot and humid climates. Thus, people in south India tend to prefer yoghurt over cheese. But paneer is a popular ingredient in north Indian dishes. According to *Bhojanakutuhalam*, paneer aggravates kapha, alleviates pitta and vāta, increases strength, and is highly recommended for those with a strong digestive fire, insomniacs and post-dalliance.

Butter is traditionally obtained by churning sour yoghurt. My mother used to set aside the creamy layer that would form on milk that had been boiled. She would do this every day for a week or so and then add a little yoghurt to the collected cream. Within a day or two, the cream would turn sour, and then she would add cold water and churn it to obtain butter. This makes more butter as the base material is mostly fat. Otherwise, one can simply churn yoghurt using a simple wooden churning rod to make fresh butter. I would demonstrate this in our cooking workshops too. Churning is a beautiful and therapeutic experience. The sound from a butter pot is like sweet music. Earlier, the bangles from my mother's hands would add to the concert. The to-and-fro motion of a churning rod enhances the prāṇa or vitality of the butter and helps balance the vāta. For example, when we use a hand fan, the alternate opposite swing of the fan balances the vāta, as the flow of air hits us in opposite directions, while the air from an unidirectional revolving electric ceiling fan hits us in one direction and can thus aggravate the vāta doṣa in us and also reduce the prāṇa-śakti.

In the same way, butter churned by hand is light, while that made by machine is low in prāṇa. Hand-churned butter is also made without heating yoghurt, while machine-produced butter may slightly heat the yoghurt. A steady churning with a wooden churning rod for fifteen to twenty minutes is also good exercise for the hand muscles and increases the mind's focus. The simple gopis of Vrindavan were expert churners. It is said that they were successful in churning Lord Krishna's heart through this simple act of churning butter.

This butter is also good for the heart. After removing the butter, what remains in the pot is called buttermilk. It's a little ironic that buttermilk has neither butter nor milk in it. It is considered one of the healthiest drinks.

To make ghee, butter is heated in a heavy and thick-bottomed pot over the fire slowly and steadily, so that all the moisture evaporates and what is left behind is golden ghee. The choice of pot is important. The heavy iron pot which retains a lot of heat can evaporate water without raising the temperature of the ghee. For ghee to taste good and last longer, one must heat it enough to remove all the moisture and at the same time not overcook it. Except for ghee, no milk or milk products, such as yoghurt, paneer/cheese, cream, butter or buttermilk can be stored at room temperature for long. So refrigeration may be handy for some time.

On the other hand, ghee that has been stored for some time has a lot of medicinal properties. For practising yogis in cold countries, ghee is a standard prescribed dairy food instead of aged, salted cheese, which is considered tāmasic. However, a body that grows up with certain food may find it difficult to gain much from a new ingredient. We will talk about this in more detail in the section on digestion.

Fresh butter or navanit is refreshing and instantly rejuvenating. It can be eaten as is, with sugar candy (misri), or served atop hot, freshly puffed rotis or a hot, mashed leafy vegetable. Butter should always be served fresh or converted into ghee within four hours of preparing it. You may ask if we can store butter in the refrigerator. The potency of the butter reduces a lot with time. Its contribution in terms of fat and vitamins will not change, but like a drug that loses potency after a certain time, the benefits of fresh butter that Ayurveda speaks of will diminish with time. So, it is better to convert it to ghee if you cannot finish it.

Fresh butter is strengthening and nourishes the tissues or dhātus. It is also cooling in potency (though yoghurt is hot), light to digest (although a fat), confers intellect, improves the complexion, curtails pitta and vāta but increases kapha, imparts taste, cures aches and pains, helps overcome fatigue, imparts lustre and is good for eye health.

Voice or speech is controlled by Udāna Vāyu—upward moving air or vāta doṣa that originates in the chest. Fresh butter or ghee checks the imbalance in this vāta and thus improves voice quality. Similarly, pitta or the fire element resides in the eye. Too much pitta can impair our vision and the strength of our eyes. Fresh butter and ghee can cool down the excess pitta in the eyes. Besides this, butter is an excellent source of vitamin A, a critical ingredient for eye health. Fresh butter from cow milk also treats bleeding disorders and that from buffalo milk is an excellent alleviator of pitta.

Buttermilk is regarded very highly in Ayurveda, like no other food. It is said that Lord Shiva drank a very deadly poison called halāhal to save all life forms and the environment. Although he was able to digest the poison, it left three marks on his divine throat. Therefore, he is popularly known by the name Nilakanṭha. One Ayurveda Ācārya proclaims, 'Looks like there was no buttermilk in Kailāsh (abode of Lord Shiva), otherwise these three marks would not have been on Shiva's throat!' The idea stems from the belief that buttermilk can heal and relieve all sorts of ailments. The following verse confirms how buttermilk balances all the three doṣas.

yathā surāṇām amṛitaṁ pradhānaṁ
tathā naraṇām bhuvi takramāḥu
amḷena vātaṁ madhureṇa pittaṁ
kaphaṁ kaṣāyeṇa nihanti sadhyaḥ

—*Bhojanakutuhalam*

Just as ambrosia is of prime importance to gods, buttermilk is important for mortals. It alleviates vāta by its sour taste, pitta by its sweet taste and kapha by its astringent taste! Different tastes or rasas have the ability to balance different doṣas (this was discussed in Section Two).

Buttermilk, white as a full moon, jasmine or a conch, has the ability to treat fever due to imbalance of vāta doṣa, jaundice (due to disturbed pitta doṣa) and abdominal disorders (gut culture). Buttermilk from cow milk treats damage caused by increase of all the three doṣas, whereas that from buffalo milk balances pitta and vāta but aggravates kapha and causes oedema (accumulation of watery fluids in cavities/tissues).

Buttermilk is prepared by adding water to yoghurt that has been churned to make butter. When the quantity of water becomes half of the churned yoghurt, that buttermilk is known as takra and considered the best. This can be drunk as it is without any additions. However, if the yoghurt is too sour, then it is best to add rock salt, roasted cumin powder, black pepper and any one fresh herb, such as coriander/cilantro leaves, curry leaves or mint leaves. Personally, I like crushed fresh curry leaves or kaffir lime leaves with white rock salt.

Buttermilk as takra has the ability to treat dysentery, anaemia (lack of sufficient red blood cells resulting in fatigue and other diseases), cardiac disorders, imbalanced vāta, urinary dysfunctions and pulmonary consumptions. One must not prescribe buttermilk when one is suffering from wounds or sores, vertigo or internal hemorrhagic disorders, and in hot summer weather and when one has suffered loss of consciousness.

Ghee is the essence of milk. After passing milk through various natural processes, what we are left with is ghee. Ghee is glorified as a rasāyana in Ayurveda because it can treat various ailments while nourishing our body in various ways. Ghee is wholesome in childhood and strengthening in youth and old age. Ghee obtained from cow milk alleviates vāta and kapha, removes fatigue and treats vitiated pitta.

Once, while cooking for a huge gathering of 4000 pilgrims, we discovered that a certain dish we had prepared was too hot and fiery. The reason was that dry red chillis more pungent/hot than the chillis prescribed in the recipe were procured by mistake. We were quite helpless at that moment, as it was too late to re-cook or recall the dish. One of the team members suggested that we add ghee because ghee counteracts the pungent taste. Though an expensive fix, we went for it as it was the only option. I remember that although the dish was still spicy, it did not affect anyone's health. The ghee had counteracted the vitiated pitta caused by the chillis.

On that day, I was reminded of Hanumanji of the great Indian epic Ramayaṇa, who, with a blazing fire on his tail, burnt the golden city of Sri Lanka, the capital of evil Ravana. Mother Sita, upon learning about the fire being set on Hanuman's tail, prayed to the fire god to protect Hanumanji's tail. The fire from Hanumanji's tail burnt all of Lanka but did not burn Hanumanji's tail. The tail was on fire but it was a cooling experience for Hanumanji. Similarly, ghee, being a fat after all, stimulates digestive fire, but balances the heat of pitta by providing a cooling effect. Fire and heat go hand in hand, yet ghee promotes one, that is, digestive fire in the stomach and counteracts/balances the other, that is, pitta doṣa in the stomach. Although there is a fire, there is a cooling effect as well.

Oil, being a fat as well, also stimulates digestive fire, but may not balance pitta. So, ghee increases digestive fire but balances vitiated pitta doṣa (agni *udipana* pitta *samana*). Ācārya Vāgabhaṭa says that the oil generally carries the property of the source it is derived from. For example, peanuts are known to increase pitta doṣa, so peanut oil will increase digestive fire, but it will not treat vitiated pitta. Rather, it will add to the problem. Peanut oil and mustard oil specifically spike pitta doṣa.

Ghee that is freshly prepared from cow's milk imparts wisdom, improves the complexion, memory, strength, retentive power and nourishment. It also cleanses the system and stabilizes the body. Ghee is thought of as life itself by scholars of the Vedas. However, ghee is mostly disapproved for children and the elderly, people who have fever and those who have very weak digestive fire (as ghee itself is fat and requires some fire to process). It is also not suited to those who have diseases caused by vitiated kapha and āma (a substance that is produced from undigested food).

4. OIL

As we briefly discussed, oil generally carries the qualities of the ingredient it is made from. Nowadays, hydrogenated vegetable fat, which is used for most packaged and ready-to-eat products, is made by blending a variety of vegetable oils, most likely to reduce the cost of production. To food industrialists, it doesn't matter which ingredient the oil is sourced from as long as it is edible.

But *Rāja Nighanṭu*, an authoritative and important lexicon (nighanṭu) of Ayurvedic drugs, cautions that one must not consume oil of unknown provenance. Different oils provide different kinds of nourishment to the body, and one needs to consume it depending on the time, place and environment.

A Brief History of Oil Production

Oil was traditionally produced by cold pressing oil seeds/nuts such as peanuts, almonds, sesame, mustard, etc., or by pressing ripened and preferably dried fruits such as coconut, olives, neem, etc. After pressing, the pulp is filtered to separate the fluid from solid pulp. The oil naturally separates from the portions that contain water. Oil produced in this way is healthy, tasty, full of nutritional value and is known as virgin oil.

Sometimes the fluid is heated over low fire to evaporate all the water to obtain pure oil.

Later, machines were used to achieve the same result. Industrial machines would leave behind perhaps 7 or 8 per cent oil in the solids. The process also required considerable horsepower and caused considerable wear and maintenance. The latest technology used to extract oil is called solvent extraction, and is now used to produce nearly 56 per cent of oil the world over. In comparison, solvent extraction removes all but about 0.5 per cent of residual oil, uses considerably less horse power, and requires less maintenance. It is relatively efficient and reliable and has low production costs.

Solvent extraction uses a chemical petroleum solvent. The most popular one is called commercial hexane. The solvent dissolves the oil and separates it from water and pulp effortlessly. To extract the oil, the seed or fruit is crushed and heated, and the solvent dissolves all of it. Later, the pulp is reheated to evaporate the solvent at 60°C and residual water at 100°C. Heating the ingredients and using the chemical results makes for an oil that isn't of very good quality. The final product is an edible oil, but the solvent is very dangerous for human health. According to the United States Environmental Protection Agency: 'Hexane is used to extract edible oils from seeds and vegetables, as a special-use solvent, and as a cleaning agent. Acute (short-term) inhalation exposure of humans to high levels of hexane causes mild central nervous system (CNS) effects, including dizziness, giddiness, slight nausea, and headache. Chronic (long term) exposure to hexane in air is associated with polyneuropathy in humans, with numbness in the extremities, muscular weakness, blurred vision, headache, and fatigue observed.'

Which Oil Is Good for Me?

Considering the toxicity of solvents used, I don't feel too comfortable using oil from such factories. After all, it's my body and my life, shouldn't I be careful what I put into it? Besides, according to Ayurveda, once an oil is heated it should be consumed and cannot be reused or reheated. That's why the oil remaining in a *kadhai* or wok after frying food is fit for nothing but external massage. So, any technique that uses a heating process during production is not conducive for consumption. Oil that is extracted using a mechanical cold press method thus tends to be better for the body. The residual oil cake retains about 7–14 per cent of the oil and is thus ideal for animal feed. In solvent extraction, the amount of oil remaining in the oil cake is barely 0.5 per cent, so the oil cake is not suitable for animal feed.

Raghunath Suri, in his classic treatise *Bhojanakutuhalam*, describes that among oils, sesame oil is the best. The Sanskrit word for oil is 'taila' and that for sesame is 'til'. This means the very word taila/oil is derived from til/sesame. So when we say oil in Ayurveda, it inherently means sesame oil. For other oils, we need to add a prefix indicating the name, such as mustard oil or coconut oil. Similarly, ghee automatically means ghee that is derived from cow milk. For any other type of ghee, we need to mention the animal's name from whose milk the ghee was made.

Sesame oil is for people of all prakṛti and can be consumed universally and at all times. It imparts beauty to the hair, is sweet, bitter and astringent in taste, hot in potency, quick to action, promotes strength, treats the vitiation of kapha and vāta, itching, wounds and improves the complexion.

I have observed that coconut oil is a very popular choice among households in southern India, while households in northern India tend to cook with mustard oil, especially in the winter. This is because coconut oil is better for warm and hot weather and mustard oil is good for consumption in cold weather. Coconut oil is cold in potency and tastes sweet. It helps gain mass (which is considered a benefit, as it is not easy to gain weight in hot weather), imparts strength, favours hair growth, alleviates pitta and vāta and may increase kapha. On the other hand, mustard oil is pungent (sharp and hot) and bitter, and hot in potency (naturally). Mustard oil can treat diseases caused by vitiated kapha and vāta, but exceedingly vitiates pitta doṣa by increasing it.

I have a pitta and kapha nature and am sensitive to food that facilitates kapha nature. Whenever I massage myself with coconut oil, I feel dull and even get a headache or body-ache. If I massage myself with mustard oil, it would increase my body temperature (pitta imbalance) and make me uncomfortable. But when I use sesame oil, which has the ability to balance the vitiation of kapha (as it is hot in potency), it always suited me. The same effects are expected when these oils are used in my diet. But my body can handle mustard oil in a cold winter.

So how do you determine the nature of the oil you use, or for that matter, any ingredient, not mentioned in Ayurvedic literature? When a fruit or vegetable grows in a climate suited to a particular doṣa, it develops the ability to counteract or balance that doṣa. For example, as coconut trees can grow in the hot climate of south India, the fruit is pitta pacifying and relieves excess heat in the body. Mustard, which grows in winter, increases pitta, that is, it has the ability to fight the chill. All vegetables that grow in winter, such as cauliflower, cabbage, etc., are high on vāta. Kapha sets in more in winter, making a person lazy. So, these vegetables, which innately fight the inertia of winter, have high vāta, which is exactly why one needs to consume them to fight the lethargy instigated by winter. This is why it is important to eat local and seasonal produce.

But remember, as these vegetables are prone to throw vāta out of balance, they need to be balanced with an appropriate amount of oil and spices, such as ginger. People of vāta nature/constitution should avoid these vegetables at night and be careful while consuming them. Similarly, coconut oil should be avoided at night as it can increase the kapha doṣa. So, we can understand the nature of an ingredient to some extent by understanding the climate it grows in, and confirm this by observing its impact on a healthy body. A healthy person is one whose doṣa nature has been in balance for a considerable period of time and they are vigilant about the impact of diet and lifestyle on the equilibrium of doṣas.

While olive oil, which comes from a fruit that grows in cold climates, is not mentioned in classic Ayurvedic literature, it is known to balance vāta doṣa but can increase kapha and pitta. So, olive oil is recommended for people who live in places with cold climates.

The following oils are listed in the *Bhojanakutuhalam* as having medicinal properties:

- Though safflower vitiates all the three doṣas, impairs nutrition, and causes itching in the eyes, it is a very good laxative and kills worms.
- Castor oil can also fight worm infestations and is a good laxative too, and it helps alleviate vāta doṣa and cure skin

disorders. It's sweet to taste and is considered a rasāyana. Castor oil instigates pitta and intensely stimulates gastric fire.

- Neem oil also is known to kill worms, alleviate kapha doṣa and treat skin disorders. Camphor oil strengthens teeth and alleviates pitta. This can be used in concoctions while brushing teeth. Oil derived from grains such as sorghum, barley and wheat alleviates all the three doṣas and is exceedingly good for the eyes. All these oils are easily available to buy.

Oil is an essential ingredient of our diet. We discussed how vegetables in general increase vāta doṣa. So, all preparations of vegetables require the use of some healthy oil or ghee. One of my favourite dishes is to steam slices of potatoes and have it with pure extra virgin olive oil (EVOO), with salt and freshly crushed pepper. Similarly, slices of steamed fresh tapioca, fresh artichoke hearts or sweet potatoes served with salt, EVOO, fresh lemon juice and fresh green chilli are really tasty.

In general, oil and ghee help keep vāta doṣa in control. Vāta doṣa, being of the air element, is extremely difficult to control and can cause a plethora of problems when out of balance—from digestive issues to a restless mind. But do note, that those with serious cardiac or similar ailments must consult doctors about their oil intake.

5. SPICES

Centuries ago, spices made their way from India all the way to northern Europe. These were traded along with luxurious items, such as silk. Sailors carried pungent peppers instead of silk and precious stones on their ships. Even today, spices are traded across continents in large and ever-growing quantities. While most people add spices to their food because they add to the flavour and enhance the taste, they play a huge role in aiding digestion (or disturbing digestion).

Years ago, black pepper was referred to as black gold. It was grown in and transported from the Malabar hills of southern India, Indonesia and neighbouring south-east Asian countries to Europe, where the price would be at par with other luxury items. Traders from the Middle East would also attribute fanciful stories to extract higher prices. It became a well-established legend that it was really a tough business to harvest the pepper from the mountains of south India. It took decades for Europeans to discover the real source and then the sea route to India, when Vasco da Gama finally arrived in Calicut on the Malabar coast. Earlier, in a failed attempt to discover India, Christopher Columbus mistook America to be India and the surrounding islands as West Indies, where he filled his ships with chilli pepper, thinking it to be black pepper. He realized his mistake after reaching Spain.

Some sources say that people would use black pepper as currency and workers' pockets in the ports of England would be sewed up to prevent them from smuggling peppercorns. These stories shouldn't surprise us, as the cost of some pure brands of saffron, in today's market, supersede the price of gold.

Apart from the monetary value, spices are priceless as they fulfil two activities that are integral to our existence—eating and digesting.

One cannot eat spices by themselves as they are either pungent or bitter. So, the combination of food and spices is very important. One needs to know the science of combining the two so as to enhance both taste and digestion.

Spice Science

Although Ayurveda encourages you to eat locally produced grains and vegetables, it recommends using spices universally. For example, although asafoetida is produced mostly in Afghanistan, you can find its use in the food of practically all the ancient temples all over India. Why so? Ācārya Vāgabhaṭa puts many spices under the category of *auṣadha varga*, which is the category of drugs or medicines. And medicines are used universally. So, all the food we consume should be local, but spices need to be global. But use of spices comes with a word of caution. Just as one should be careful to regulate the doses of medicines, one should be mindful of the quantity of spices that are being consumed.

Vegetables and grains found locally are generally conducive to people who are accustomed to the climate. But the individual tridoṣa prakṛti varies from person to person, and to make sure the locally available ingredients agree with the individual, one needs to use spices. They not only help with digestion but also enhance the appearance, fragrance and taste of the food. When used properly, spices stimulate the secretion of bile and enzymes in the mouth and stomach, balance the tridoṣa disturbances caused by grains or vegetables and treat many anomalies in the body, such as purifying blood to improve the health of pancreas, liver, etc.

Those who have kapha prakṛti need to add hot spices, such as black pepper, to stimulate the digestive fire; those with pitta prominence in their nature need cooling spices, such as clove, and those with vāta as the prominent doṣa need to use a combination of hot and cool spices to avoid aggravation of vāta.

Similarly, ingredients that have more kapha need hot spices, pitta-dominant food needs cooling spices and vāta ingredients need a combination of both. However, spices are more than just balancing kapha, vāta or pitta.

Every spice is unique in its fragrance and has numerous medicinal properties. To use it precisely to enhance the taste, look, texture and experience of eating, one needs training from expert cooks. Usually, like many other traditions in India, older members of families possess deep knowledge about culinary concepts, which is passed on from generation to generation. Now this science is neither taught nor encouraged in the universities of modern education. Even in hotel management colleges or home science departments, the focus has unfortunately shifted away from these traditions. Though some books remain, they are in languages unknown to modern students. And those who understand it lack tradition and experience. But fortunately, the science of spices still exists in many Vedic temples all over India. From these temple recipes, which mainly cook sāttvic food following Ayurvedic principles, we can look into the appropriate use of spices, especially pertaining to local climate. Thus, while many spices may balance kapha and vāta doṣas, only specific ones are used according to the ingredient and preparation, keeping in mind factors such as taste, fragrance and medicinal impacts. In the following discussion, we will examine the characteristics of each spice as well as the accompanying tradition.

We will discuss essential spices (like asafoetida, black pepper, cumin, mustard, coriander, clove, cinnamon, ginger) and different types of salt.

Asafoetida (Hingu): This ingredient is used in almost all Ayurvedic preparations of vegetables and soups from lentils. Asafoetida is known to aggravate pitta (thus increasing the strength of gastric fire) and balances kapha and vāta. It is a sāttvic ingredient, although many Hatha yogis avoid it as it is known to subtly stimulate the nervous system. But it's an important ingredient from the purview of Ayurveda principles as it aids digestion and balances vāta (thus bloating, etc). As Ayurveda's primary concern is to lengthen one's life span, it supports anything that promotes life.

I found that asafoetida is used in all centuries-old traditional Vaishnava temples throughout India (Vishnu is considered the Lord of sattva guṇa). Most of these temples still follow age-old cooking techniques. Notably, in Jagannath Puri, the cooks still use clay pots and cook over a wood fire. They are particular about using locally grown grains and vegetables, which means you won't find fresh green chilli, potatoes or tomatoes in that kitchen. In fact, they call tomato 'bilāyati bāingan', which means 'eggplant from England'. There are striking similarities between the tomato plant and eggplant. But when the tomato plant fructifies, the fruit is reddish, resembling the colour of an Englishman, hence the name.

Despite being so strict about following local traditions, the cooks of Jagannath Puri use asafoetida profusely, which grows mostly in Afghanistan. This proves how the use of spice indeed is global.

When used appropriately, asafoetida increases the perception of taste and thus helps in digestion from the very beginning. Ayurveda prescribes cooking asafoetida in ghee and then adding the vegetables or protein to it.

Asafoetida is a solidified tree sap and is technically a resin. It is very hard and has a strong odour. Pots containing pure asafoetida carry the fragrance for a very long time, making them unfit to store anything else. Most of the asafoetida that is now available is mixed with flour, and needs to be used with caution. The grains are mixed to ease the pounding and processing of hard resins of asafoetida. I always add this powder directly to hot ghee or oil and ensure that it is cooked well before it mixes with the other ingredients. The ghee should be moderately hot just so that it can cook the asafoetida. Upon contact with ghee the asafoetida slowly turns brown and emanates a nice aroma. Otherwise, if uncooked, the strong raw odour may manifest in the cooked food and disturb the taste. But overcooking the spice over high heat will rid it of all its essential qualities. If you are using the solid resin, use a sturdy metal pestle and mortar to pound it into small particles before adding it to hot ghee. Please refer to the recipes in Section Five for more details on how to use it.

Black Pepper (Marica): This universal spice is a wonder in itself. It balances kapha and vāta doṣas. It is light to digest as it is pungent in taste and fiery in nature. It is well suited to cold climates, such as countries in Europe, but because it is easily digested, it is also found in the recipes prepared in the hot climate of central and southern India.

Though it enhances digestive power, it does not cause acidity or heartburn. To me, it is an ideal spice, as it adds to taste, helps with the digestion of grains and vegetables, and does not add to the stomach's load. Chilli pepper/hot green chilli (which was brought by Columbus to Europe) can increase digestive power because of its hot potency and has properties similar to black pepper but is less effective in balancing vāta as it causes dryness. So chilli pepper should be consumed with care. Although black pepper is pungent, it does not cause a burning sensation, whereas chilli pepper does. One should gradually try to replace chilli pepper (fresh or dried) with black pepper.

Ayurveda says black pepper is used to cure many ailments, such as worm infestations and is especially effective in fighting cold, cough and throat infections. If you feel a throat infection coming on, take two pepper corns, a clove and a small chunk of rock sugar candy (khadi sakar) and slowly press them all between your teeth while sucking on the essence for ten to fifteen minutes. It will greatly relieve the symptoms and likely cure the infection too.

A few pinches of freshly crushed black pepper with honey also treats cold. It also enhances the voice, and many classical singers use it to improve and maintain their voice quality. However, too much black pepper can make food rājasic (enjoyment at the cost of health) and tāmasic (destruction of health). So, although black pepper and chilli pepper have similar impacts on doṣas, black pepper has more medicinal attributes.

Ginger (Adraka and Sunthi): This is yet another useful spice in the family of hot pungent spices. Both fresh as well as dried ginger have the same health benefits. This root mitigates kapha and vāta and increases pitta. It is an excellent spice to kindle the digestive fire. Black pepper is more aggressive, in the sense that the after-effect is pungent too, whereas that of ginger is sweet. That means that although ginger is pungent on the tongue, the taste becomes sweet after being digested.

So, ginger is less likely to cause acidity or heartburn. On top of that, it balances vāta, which means it will prevent bloating. Black pepper doesn't cause a burning sensation either, for it is easier to digest. But yet, one cannot add too much black pepper. One can increase the amount of ginger in a dish without a hitch. Despite all these advantages, I don't see ginger used much in south India, or as much as it is in north and central India. The preferred spice in the region is pepper, better suited to the hot climate of the south. Some recipes use ginger, especially those with sprouts as the major ingredient. Some also use ginger in curd rice and buttermilk.

Ginger must be added to heavy food, such as lentils, soaked chickpeas and kidney beans (chole and rajma). The quantity of ginger should increase in proportion to the heaviness of the ingredients and dish preparation. For example, chickpeas require almost three times the quantity of ginger that moong beans do.

Ginger is not prominent in European cuisines, probably because it was difficult to transport fresh ginger, and dried ginger is mostly used as medicines and difficult to produce and trade. Black pepper, however, was handy for the traders and did not spoil easily.

On the other hand, Chinese cuisines value ginger as highly as pepper. Unfortunately, in India, chilli pepper is used in recipes that would originally call for black pepper and ginger, whereas Chinese and European cuisines still prefer pepper and ginger as the key pungent spice.

Ginger also counters weight gain, indigestion, cough and dyspnoea (difficulty in breathing) and relieves constipation. It adds taste to the food and helps with the absorption of water in the body (helps hydration). Ginger tea is very effective in relieving cold and cough. Just boil with water and jaggery.

There are a few more pungent spices (such as long pepper or pippali), but Ācārya Vāgabhaṭa does not encourage their use in cooking, but only as medicines.

The three spices we have discussed are a source of fire and lead to digestion in a very controlled environment of the stomach. But this fire also needs to be moderated. So, many cooling spices and herbs are added at the right time and in appropriate quantities. We will discuss a few such spices.

Cinnamon (Dalcini): Cinnamon bark is pungent in taste but is cooling in potency and light or easy to digest. It treats the vitiation of kapha and thus helps cleanse the throat. Cinnamon leaf or bay leaf is hot as well as cold! It can treat the vitiation of kapha and vāta. Cinnamon is added to food that is heavy to digest, such as Bengal gram (chana dal or kala chana or split baby chickpeas), chickpeas, raw jackfruit (kathhal), etc. It is also used in sambar masala. The basic contribution of this spice is to balance the heat of spices, such as pepper and ginger, and yet not counteract them as this spice is pungent itself.

Clove (Lavang): Clove is bitter and cooling. It is used along with cinnamon, but because it has a bitter taste, it should be used sparingly. The main advantage of this spice, however, is in its ability to treat vitiation of all the three doṣas. Clove is good for the eyes, cures diseases of the head and imparts taste to food. Clove with cinnamon and bay leaf is especially used to flavour pulao. If used in the right proportion and cooked correctly, the fragrance of a pulao can charm one's mind and satisfy one's heart completely. But care must be taken not to bite into the clove or any of these spices directly as they are mostly pungent or bitter in taste. Some suggest grinding these spices before adding, but that may affect the overall taste as the spices are generally pungent and bitter. Only spices such as cumin, fennel and coriander are to be used in powdered form while cooking. Cinnamon and clove are also good for dental health and counter bad breath. Sucking on tiny pieces of these spices is the right way to improve oral health.

Cardamom (Elaichi): There are two types of cardamom. The popular one is the green/white variety with small seeds, while the black one has larger seeds (badi elaichi). While both green and black varieties are capable of balancing kapha and vāta, the black one increases pitta. The green one is cold in potency while the black variety is hot. Green cardamom is added to milk to balance kapha and vāta, but not black cardamom. The latter is useful in improving digestive fire but at the same time balancing vāta, for example, while cooking chickpeas or kidney beans. Green cardamom is easy to digest whereas black elaichi is pungent after digestion. The green variety will have cooling properties and can help ease heartburn and a burning sensation during urination and itching. On the other hand, black cardamom, which increases pitta, is likely to aggravate these problems. Both impart a nice fragrance to the mouth, fight cough and improve intellect, but should be avoided during pregnancy. Cardamom pods are bitter, so care must be taken not to bite into them directly.

It is a common practice to use spices, such as black pepper, cinnamon, clove and cardamom in sweets, as these are known to reduce kapha doṣa. For example, the famous laddus of

Tirupati Balaji, which are made from chickpea flour, have plenty of green cardamoms in it. The cooks of Jagannath Puri use the seeds of black elaichi in the preparation of laddus made from wholewheat flour and clove powder in the preparation of khaja (which is similar to baklava).

Carom (Yavani or Ajwain): Carom seeds or bishop seeds are pungent and bitter. They are highly effective for soothing stomach disorders. They provide quick relief from indigestion and gas. For quick relief, it is best to drink water that ajwain has been soaked in. Or just crush half/quarter of a teaspoon of ajwain with a mortar and pestle, and drink it with warm water. It provides relief within an hour and helps rekindle the digestive fire. This spice is used to cook with heavy food, such as chickpeas, or dishes that use chickpea flour or white flour (pakoras/savouries like samosa, kadhi, etc.). It treats disorders in the kapha and vāta doṣas.

Fenugreek (Methi): Fenugreek seeds are very useful in bringing down excess vāta and kapha. This is used especially to balance the sour taste of kapha-dominant food, for example sambar (south Indian lentil soup with some assorted vegetables). Similarly, sour fermented food (like dosa, idlis which are prepared from fermented batter of urad dal/black gram and rice) of south India, preparations from yoghurt (like kadhi) in northern India, also require fenugreek to help smooth digestion. In eastern India, cooks use fenugreek while cooking with sour ingredients, called 'khatā' from raw mango or tamarind. So, if you are cooking with anything sour, make sure to add fenugreek seeds. It also increases the digestive fire and appetite. Fried fenugreek seeds taste great too. It is especially effective in controlling gastritis and bloating. Idlis and dosas for example can significantly cause bloating without methi. It is full of vitamins and easily available. Fenugreek, known as methika in Sanskrit, is known to increase medha or intelligence and knowledge. A half teaspoon of soaked methi boiled with milk can be served with jaggery to lactating mothers to increase production of breast milk. However, one should avoid use of methi in case of anal or nasal bleeding.

Mustard (Sarson/Rai): Seeds from mustard plants are used widely in Indian cuisine. This pungent spice is hot in potency and mitigates vāta and kapha while it increases pitta. It is usually used with a combination of cooling spices, such as fennel. Mustard paste is used as a condiment in many dishes. But usually, it needs to be moderated by some cooling spice. For example, in Jagannath Puri, they cook a dish called Besar, which combines mustard and fennel paste. Mustard paste is also used by Bengalis in a bitter dish called Sukto, but the taste is moderated by the use of poppy seeds which are cool in potency. Mustard has a unique sharp taste and helps reduce itching.

Cumin (Jeera): This spice is also pungent, enhances taste considerably, is hot in potency and increases pitta, thus aiding in digestion, and balances kapha and vāta. This spice is also used across India. It is light to digest, but has an effect similar to mustard. The pitta-increasing effect of cumin is moderated by frying it in ghee. Roasted cumin powder is used in many preparations. Whether in buttermilk or lentil soups, it immensely enhances the taste and reduces the effect of kapha in buttermilk and vāta in lentil preparations.

Coriander/Cilantro Seeds or Leaves (Dhania): This is one of the rare spices that is sweet after digestion, so it is considered excellent for balancing pitta. It balances vāta as it is hot in potency and balances kapha as it is bitter and astringent in taste. In other words it balances all the three doṣas. This spice is used a lot in south India, where the climate and food is likely to cause pitta imbalance. The leaves have similar properties, so they can be used for everything except sweets.

Turmeric (Haldi): This spice has steadily been gaining the world's attention. It is a fascinating spice in the sense that apart from balancing all the three doṣas, it carries more than twenty medicinal properties to fight various diseases. It particularly facilitates efficient liver function, purification of the blood, intestine tract and skin. According to Cancer Research UK, laboratory studies on cancer cells have shown that curcumin, a compound found in turmeric, has anti-cancer effects. It seems to be able to kill cancer cells and prevent more from growing. It has the most impact on breast cancer, bowel cancer, stomach cancer and skin cancer cells. Naturally, if included in our daily diet, it can protect us from many diseases.

Turmeric is pungent and bitter and hot in potency. The hot potency due to pungent taste balances kapha and vāta doṣa. The bitterness is helpful for balancing pitta doṣa. We have discussed the relationship between taste and doṣa in detail in Section Two of this book. For culinary purposes, it is mostly used in its powdered form and preserves all medicinal properties when cooked with boiling vegetables or grains. It can even be cooked in ghee over a low flame. If it is to be added to a tadka (tempering), it is better to do so after adding wet spices, such as ginger paste. This norm should be followed for all ground spices, except for asafoetida (which is a tree sap).

Fennel (Sounf): This is perhaps the only spice that tastes sweet. It has a similar effect as cumin and is normally served after finishing the meal to keep the mouth fresh and hydrated. It also helps in digestion, but is not advised for people facing difficulty in procreation. However, it is safe to consume during pregnancy. Fennel is also used in many sweet preparations like mālpoa, as it adds a sweet fragrance and helps with digestion.

Saffron (Kesar): Saffron is a luxury spice found in very unique cold climates, such as that of the Himalayas. The fragrance of saffron is divinely intoxicating (but does not cause a high or low in the mood). The high cost is associated with its low production rate and difficulty in harvesting it. It is hot in potency, and bitter and pungent in taste. So, it balances the kapha and vāta doṣas of the ingredients when it is added to, milk for example. Around eight to ten threads of saffron are sufficient for two cups of milk. Saffron with a pod of green cardamom (thrashed) and a teaspoon of sugar candy makes milk taste heavenly. Saffron also cures disorders of the throat, stimulates digestive fire and improves complexion. I use saffron on festive occasions, specially while cooking vegetable pulao, risotto, ras malai, mālpoa, sweet rice, modak and gulab jamun.

Camphor (Karpura): Edible camphor, which is derived from the camphor tree (found in the Himalayas) is cold in potency and treats vitiation of kapha and bleeding disorders (imbalance of pitta). Pinches of camphor relax the eyes and have a cooling effect on them. Camphor is used mostly to cook sweets, adding a subtle divine taste that cannot be described in words, and is considered auspicious. Saffron and camphor when added in the right quantities to sweet rice (prepared from milk, rice and rock sugar candy) make it taste heavenly. Camphor is used in Tirupati Balaji's Laddu Prasadam. Care must be taken to discriminate between chemical camphor (naphtha balls) and naturally harvested camphor. Even a little extra camphor will make the preparation bitter.

Musk (Kasturi): Musk is generated in the glands of the musk deer in the region of the navel. It should only be obtained from a musk deer that has died naturally. It is very expensive. Its fragrance is unparalleled, and ancient texts say that the poor deer itself runs hither thither to determine the source of this intoxicating smell. This is an analogy to understand that all the great wealth of happiness lies within ourselves, so instead of looking for it outside, we should look within our own self. Otherwise, like the deer, one eventually dies searching for it with sadness all his/her life.

This intoxicating fragrance is considered an auspicious offering for gods and kings. Earlier, specially trained chefs used this in culinary preparations for the enjoyment of the kings. But (thankfully though), that use is extinct now.

Salt: Spice and salt go hand in hand. A great Vaishnava saint once said that a man should be like salt—his presence should not be conspicuous, and he should serve without worrying about the results. On the other hand, spices are praised even if they are subtly present. But salt is not to be discounted, as when it is absent, no one speaks of the spices but sorely misses the salt.

But salt doesn't just play the role of a taste enhancer. In general, salt increases digestion and the perception of taste, mitigates vāta and kapha, and aggravates pitta. It is useful in clearing bowels. Different types of salt vary slightly in their properties. Saindhava lavaṇa, which is also known as rock salt, and Himalayan salt, is the best according to Ācārya Vāgabhaṭa. It is successful in mitigating pitta doṣa as it is cold in potency, and thus it balances all the three doṣas. This salt comes in two colours, white and pink. White is considered superior. Saindhava salt is the only salt that is good for eyes. It is found in the Sindh region of Punjab (far from the Himalayas) in Pakistan.

Once, there used to be a huge ocean in the region that dried out, leaving behind pure crystals of mineral salt. Note the power of vāta doṣa (air and ether elements). If vāta can dry an ocean, think of how much it can dry our bodies. Dryness of skin is a result of aggravated vāta. Salt that is completely dried out by air attracts water and thus is a natural antidote for vāta. Oil prevents loss of water while salt attracts water. This is indicated by the thirst we experience on consuming something that is salty. This property empowers salt to mitigate vāta. But there is a contraindication too. Excessive salt may increase the water retention in the body, thus increasing blood pressure. High blood pressure, when unchecked, can lead to brain strokes and heart failures. Thus, it is important to moderate the amount of salt used in cooking and consumption.

Sea salt that is harvested in clean lands and has traces of minerals is considered good for health. Harvested sea salt stimulates digestive fire and imparts taste. Compared with other salts, it does not cause much pitta disturbance (and hence does not cause burning sensation and skin disorders) as it is slightly sweet in taste. It balances kapha and vāta in the abdomen. However, *Bhojanakutuhalam* says that sea salt can cause greying of hair and vitiation of blood, causing burning sensation.

Black salt, which is mined in the Kangra district of Himachal Pradesh, has a high content of iron and sulphur. It is used in vegan food to replicate the sulphide smell of eggs. It is the main ingredient in chat masala, along with dried mango powder which gives it that special taste. This salt is good for mitigating indigestion and should be consumed when one has fever. Black salt when combined with carom seeds (ajwain) relieves bloating and gas effectively.

Salt that is refined in factories and fortified with iodine is called table salt. Refined salt is bereft of many essential minerals that naturally harvested salt has. Around fifty to eighty-four trace minerals naturally occur in the salt. Some of these bonus minerals include: calcium, potassium, sulphur, magnesium, iron, phosphorus, iodine, manganese, copper, zinc and dozens more. Table salt has only two elements—sodium and chloride. All other minerals are removed as 'impurities' during the refining process. So without a doubt, look for unrefined harvested salt or mined salt like Himalayan pink salt or saindha salt.

How does one determine how much salt should be added to food? I suggest keeping a standard spoon, say the size of a half teaspoon, and adding measured quantities while cooking. If it goes wrong, then you know how much to adjust next time you cook the recipe. It's tough to adjust the salt when you add it by approximation. For reference, in general, a litre or 4 cups

(4.3 American cups) of any cooked product requires nearly a teaspoon of saindha salt.

Table 3.4 summarizes the impact of spices on tridoṣa. The up arrow indicates an increase in that doṣa and the down arrow indicates that it balances that doṣa, especially if it is disturbed. This table will be helpful while charting your own diet plan. For example, a pitta prakṛti person should use pitta-increasing spices in moderation, while a person of kapha prakṛti may use more of a spice that balances kapha. Similarly, if an ingredient has more vāta in it, say potato, then we should cook it with more of a vāta-calming spice, such as ginger.

Table 3.4: Properties of Spices

Spices	Taste: Before & After Digestion	Potency	Impact on Tridoṣa	Important for Persons with
Asafoetida	B: Pungent A: Pungent	Hot and Easy to digest	K↓V↓P↑	Vāta Prakṛti
Black Pepper	B: Pungent A: Pungent	Hot and Easy to digest	K↓V↓	Kapha & Vāta Prakṛti
Ginger	B: Pungent A: Sweet	Hot and Easy to digest	K↓V↓P↑	Kapha & Vāta Prakṛti
Cumin	B: Pungent A: Sweet	Hot and Easy to digest	K↓V↓P↑	For all
Coriander	B: Pungent A: Sweet	Hot and Easy to digest	K↓V↓P↓	For all
Fennel	B: Sweet A: Sweet	Hot and Easy to digest	K↓V↓	For all

Mustard	B: Pungent A: Pungent	Hot and easy to digest	K↓V↓P↑	Kapha & Vāta Prakṛti
Chilli pepper	B: Pungent A: Pungent	Hot and Easy to digest	K↓V↓P↑	Kapha & Vāta Prakṛti
Fenugreek	B: Bitter A: Pungent	Hot and Easy to digest	K↓V↓	For all
Turmeric	B: Bitter A: Pungent	Hot and Easy to digest	K↓V↓P↓	For all
Cinnamon	B: Pungent, sweet A: Pungent	Cold and easy to digest	K↓V↓P↑	Kapha & Vāta Prakṛti
Clove	B: Bitter A: Pungent	Cold and easy to digest	K↓V↓P↓	For all
Cardamom	B: Pungent, sweet A: Pungent	Cold	K↓V↓	For all
Saffron	B: Bitter A: Pungent	Hot and easy to digest	K↓V↓P↓	For all
Saindha Salt	B: Salty A: salty	Cold	K↓V↓P↓	For all
Carom	B: Bitter A: Pungent	Cold and easy to digest	K↓V↓P↑	For all

6. FRUITS

Generally there is a misconception that fruits are not be mixed or had with cooked food. Such rules are not found in Ayurvedic texts. Traditionally, we have seen bananas being a part of meals in south India. Mangoes are eaten after a full meal all over India, and coconut chutney is offered with idlis and dosas. So, four major fruits—banana, mango, coconut and jackfruit—are eaten along with the meal. All fruits can be similarly combined with a meal if it does not break other rules mentioned in Viruddha Āhāra (incompatible foods), which is discussed in the next section. The general rule is that heavy food be eaten first and light food towards the end of the meal. Consumption of fruits follows the same rule.

Can fruits be eaten by themselves? Yes, but in general, there should be a gap of four to five hours between two meals to allow the previous meal to be digested completely. Ayurveda does not encourage eating at night, especially fruits, as they increase kapha and, in general, are heavy to digest. If you eat two meals a day, there is no choice but to eat fruits during the meal or make one meal entirely of fruits. I have seen my revered Gurudev follow the latter rule for years.

Fruits are often combined with dairy products, such as custard. Ayurveda does not deem that problematic, unless the combination is completely unsuitable. For example, it is not a good idea to mix sour fruits with milk.

Sour fruits can go well with yoghurt but may disturb pitta doṣa to a large extent. Yoghurt itself is heavy and requires a good digestive capacity to process it. So, it is important to eat it at a time when the digestive fire is high. One must also be careful while sweetening yoghurt. For example, honey and yoghurt don't go together (when combined in equal proportions). It is best to use rock sugar candy pounded into a powder.

Before we discuss specific fruits, it is important to know that most fruit is available in a variety of tastes. For example, grapes can be sour or sweet. The sweet variety of the same fruit acts on our tridoṣa differently from the sour variety. So, care must be taken while purchasing the product. Recently, I was in Bologna, Italy, where we visited a fruit vendor, who was happily passing around samples of his fruit before we made a decision. In an ideal scenario, it would be best to sample the fruit before you buy it, but this is often not possible, so make sure you have a fruit vendor you can trust.

Grapes: 'Drakshā phalottamā', of all fruits, Ayurveda considers grapes the best. Ripened sweet grapes are cold in potency and balance kapha and vāta. This fruit is full of nutrition, improves the power of the voice and throat, is good for the eyes, relieves coughs and is known to be a very good cleansing agent and thus helpful in clearing bowels. Grapes are very good for cardiac health too. Dried grapes/raisins are known to mitigate excessive thirst, dryness and excessive burning sensation. It is also soothing to have it after vomiting.

Grapes can even help with hangovers and in de-addiction. Raisins calm the mind too. Grapes go well with pomegranate and dates. This fruit is prone to be attacked by pests and so may come to the market loaded with pesticides. So, care must be taken to find organic grapes. In any case, wash the fruit/raisins several times before consuming. Raisins soaked in water for three to four hours balance pitta and relieve gastric problems. It is a good habit to consume eight to ten raisins (soaked overnight) early in the morning on an empty stomach.

Fully ripened sour grapes are very effective for treating vāta imbalance but increase kapha and pitta. Unripe sour grapes are hot in potency and cause skin rashes, whereas ripened grapes are considered healthy and calm pitta, apart from balancing kapha and vāta.

Banana: A naturally ripe banana is a true delight. There are many varieties of bananas, and some are full of aroma and flavour. It is considered as a deva-fruit, one that is fit for gods and is offered in temples across India. The other three fruits in this category are coconut, mango and jackfruit. Bananas are very good for balancing pitta and vāta, but increase kapha. So, bananas are eaten at the end of a meal to take care of acidity/pitta caused by excessive spices. People of kapha prakṛti, especially with a low digestive fire, will find it difficult to eat bananas as it aggravates the kapha doṣa and is heavy to digest. This effect is usually mitigated by combining it with black pepper and camphor.

Milk and banana can be combined only when the banana is ripened well through natural means, and there is no sourness in the fruit. One should avoid eating bananas at night and very early in the morning, as kapha tends to aggravate due to the cooler temperature during this period and because bananas are heavy to digest. When mature and ripened, bananas are sweet and slightly astringent. They instantly increase virility, banish thirst and provide strength. Yellow fragrant ripe bananas are the best kind, followed by the dark red variety.

Banana is a rich source of vitamin B6 and has no fat. It regulates blood sugar by providing soluble fibre in the blood stream and helps to keep the kidneys clean. Vitamin B6 plays a vital role in boosting the metabolism and soothing the nervous system.

Pomegranate: Pomegranates come in two varieties—sweet and sour. The sweet variety balances all the three doṣas while the sour kind balances kapha and vāta but increases pitta. Only very sweet fruits are capable of balancing all the three doṣas. Pomegranate has three distinct tastes, sweet, sour and astringent, which helps to take care of the imbalances of the three doṣas. Unfortunately, this fruit also tends to absorb a lot of pesticides, so we must be careful about the source and wash it several times before eating.

Pomegranates can be eaten at any time of the day. It is light in potency and easily digested and wholesome. It is highly recommended in times of illness, nausea and diarrhoea. However, it can cause constipation.

Coconut: Coconut is not a nut but a fruit. People often mistake it for a nut because of its hard protective shell. The pulp is sweet and helps one gain weight. It is heavy to digest, cold in potency and balances vāta and pitta doṣas. It also cleanses and detoxifies the urinary tract. Tender coconut water is easy to digest, relieves excess heat in the body quickly and is an excellent diuretic too. Mature coconut water is heavy to digest, but slightly balances pitta doṣa. Coconut milk has properties similar to coconut and works as a good cardiac tonic, whereas coconut oil is not conducive for heart health. Dried coconut (kopra) is heavy and difficult to digest and causes a burning sensation, but augments strength and virility. So, it must be eaten with cooling spices, such as cinnamon and clove.

7. WATER (APAḤ)

Lord Krishna says in the Bhagavad Gitā, 'Of all the drinks, I am the taste of water'. No liquids can quench one's thirst like water. Nor can anyone replace water. Water symbolizes purity; not only does it remove dirt but it also purifies the mind. The quality of water is determined by its source.

Pure water (100 per cent H_2O) without minerals is considered unhealthy as it extracts stored minerals from our body through reverse osmosis. Interestingly, this same reverse osmosis (RO-water) technique is used to remove unwanted particles from water to purify it. Many years ago, we installed one RO unit in our ashram to provide clean water especially for the visiting guests from western countries with sensitive alimentary canals. But we realized the inmates' health was getting adversely affected. A simple test showed that RO water is not only bereft of essential minerals but also found to be slightly acidic! We disconnected the unit and used a normal filter.

Terrestrial water sources are rivers, lakes, wells and ponds. Water found in deserts is considered very beneficial, cures several diseases, stimulates digestive fire and is light to digest. Such water aggravates kapha and is slightly salty. Water collected from marshy land or areas surrounded by a thick growth of trees aggravates vāta and should not be consumed as it can cause several diseases. But water from land that is neither a desert nor marshy is sweet, cooling in potency, light to digest and balances all three doṣas. It nourishes all the tissues and imparts taste. The taste of cooked food depends on the source of water. I know of catering companies in Amritsar that order special tankers of water to ensure good taste.

Water from rivers varies due to their geographical positions. Of all the rivers in India, Gangā is considered the best by the Ayurvedic Ācāryas and the next is Godāvari. Nowadays, by the time these rivers reach the plains, the water is heavily polluted. This reminds me of Ācārya Vāgabhaṭa warning that one should be aware of the qualities of water one drinks and uses for cooking purposes.

MEAT PRODUCTS

Meat products, although tāmasic, are extensively discussed in classic Ayurvedic texts. One reason is that there are places on our planet where no vegetation grows in certain seasons. Ayurveda's purpose is to nourish and preserve the human form of life. Ayurveda describes in great detail how meat should be cooked and eaten in ways that imparts health and long life.

According to Ayurveda, meat is a natural food for human consumption, but utmost care needs to be taken while handling it, as it easily gets contaminated. So, there are detailed descriptions on each type of meat, the impact on tridoṣa and cooking methods for appropriate digestion. However, we will forgo the detailed discussion of each type of meat as this book focuses on the importance of sāttvic food in our lives.

Designing Your Food Profile

In this section we discussed the importance of sāttvic food in promoting health and peace of mind. We also discussed the triguṇa nature of various food ingredients. Now, using all this information, we will attempt to make a sāttvic food profile for various prakṛti. Follow these steps to design your food profile.

1. From Section One, estimate your triguṇa nature. Depending on your triguṇa nature, you need to create your sāttvic diet. If you are involved in a lot of intellectual activity, then your sāttvic diet will include light meals of grains, vegetables, legumes and dairy products. If your activities involve physical labour, then include heavy meals in your diet, comprising legumes and proteins (like cheese) along with grains and vegetables. You may also have to eat more than someone who is mainly involved in intellectual work. Eat till the hunger is satisfied.
2. From Section One, find out your tridoṣa prakṛti. This will help you further refine your sāttvic diet. For example, Table 3.4 summarized the properties of some prominent spices. You will find how each spice is linked to various doṣa prakṛti. See how to combine them in a way that

preserves your tridoṣa constitution. Below, Table 3.5 summarizes the use of spices and some prominent ingredients for people with various prakṛti. These are some basic rules to be followed while cooking the ingredients. Always keep in mind that the prakṛti of the food needs to include food/spices that are opposite to the nature of a person consuming it to maintain the equilibrium of the doṣas. This is generally achieved through using proper spices while using an ingredient of the same nature as yours. Or, use a food ingredient of the opposite nature directly. For example, if you are of kapha nature, then you will naturally be attracted to earthy wholesome food like potatoes or cheese. Use enough ginger and black pepper to calm down the kapha-aggravating nature of these food ingredients. Or, use food ingredients with less kapha nature in it like bottle gourd (lauki). A person of kapha prakṛti will be attracted to food of kapha nature, consumption of which may increase that doṣa. So, one needs to learn the correct cooking procedures to derive the maximum benefits while maintaining the doṣa equilibrium.

Table 3.5: Combining Spices and Food

Your Prakṛti ➡ Ingredient ⬇	**Kapha or kapha as prominent Prakṛti**	**Pitta or pitta as prominent Prakṛti**	**Vāta or vāta as prominent Prakṛti**
Moong dal K↑P↓V↓	Use ginger, pepper and ghee/ oil.	Use asafoetida, ginger and ghee.	Use extra ghee, a little ginger and lemon.

Your Prakṛti ➡ Ingredient ↓	Kapha or kapha as prominent Prakṛti	Pitta or pitta as prominent Prakṛti	Vāta or vāta as prominent Prakṛti
Pigeon pea (toor dal) K↓P↓V↑	Use ginger, pepper and ghee.	Use asafoetida, ginger and ghee.	Use extra ghee, a little ginger and lemon.
Bengal gram (chana dal) K↓P↑V↑	Use ginger, pepper and ghee and cooling spices like clove and cinnamon.	Use asafoetida, cumin and coriander powder, ginger, ghee, cooling spices like clove and cinnamon, herbs like coriander.	Use extra ghee, ginger, lemon and asafoetida.
Chickpea (chole) K↓P↑V↑	Use more ginger, pepper and ghee/oil and less cooling spices like clove, cinnamon and bay leaf.	Same as above but more cooling spices, and topped with more ghee and fresh mint.	Avoid excess ginger but add more ghee and asafoetida.
Root Veggies K↓P↑V↑	Use more ginger, pepper and (mustard) oil and less cooling spices like clove, cinnamon and bay leaf.	Same as above but more cooling spices, and topped with more ghee and fresh mint.	Avoid excess ginger, ghee and asafoetida.
Milk K↑P↓V↑	Saffron, cardamom, ginger powder	Saffron, cardamom	Saffron
Fresh Yoghurt K↑P↑V↑	Cumin powder, ginger, coriander leaves	Cumin powder, black pepper, mint	Asafoetida, coriander leaves

Your Prakṛti ➡ Ingredient ⬇	**Kapha or kapha as prominent Prakṛti**	**Pitta or pitta as prominent Prakṛti**	**Vāta or vāta as prominent Prakṛti**
Fresh Cheese	Use more ginger, pepper and ghee/oil and less cooling spices like clove, cinnamon and bay leaf.	Use asafoetida, cumin and coriander powder, ginger, ghee, less cooling spices like clove and cinnamon, herbs like coriander.	Use extra ghee, ginger, lemon and asafoetida.
↓↑moderately low or high	**↑↓Too high or low**	**↓↑ Mild influence**	

3. Determine a proper quantity for consumption. Because of low digestive fire in kapha prakṛti people, it is difficult to decide when to stop eating, thus leading to eating disorders. In case of pitta prakṛti, because of increased hunger, they know exactly when the hunger is satisfied, and thus refrain from eating. In case of vāta prakṛti, it could be either, as vāta could either increase the fire or reduce it. If you have ever cooked on a wood fire stove, you can easily relate to this. High wind sometimes extinguishes the wood fire, while a steady flow of air builds up the fire to a point that even a heavy flow of breeze cannot extinguish the fire. I have discussed this elaborately in the following Section describing digestion. One needs to be mindful of this.
4. Plan a proper menu. The next section will help you decide on a proper menu which depends upon the time (breakfast/lunch/dinner and season), place (desert, snow, etc.) and proper combination of food. You need

to understand which food preparations go together to nourish and which do not.

5. Cook in adherence to the principles of Ayurveda. This is also described in detail in this section as well as in Section Five. I have seen how cooks in many traditional temples take a lot of care while cooking, because they can't afford to make mistakes when they cook for gods. So, the menu, the recipes and Ayurvedic knowledge are still intact in their cooking. I have included a few recipes in this book in Section Five. Someday, I dream of putting all those recipes together in another book with Ayurvedic explanations. At the moment, I try to pass on as much knowledge as possible in my workshops.

Conclusion

Of all the foods, according to Ayurveda, sāttvic food is the best and it needs to be fine-tuned to our unique nature. But what if the person himself/herself is not fit? What if they eat the right thing at the wrong time? What if they eat the wrong quantity? What if they are stressed, distressed, dejected or depressed? Even if we are able to cook good food, following Ayurvedic principles, it will not nourish us correctly if we cannot digest it. Of course, there is more to our nature than just triguṇa and tridoṣa. These two aspects form our fundamental nature. But, for proper digestion and assimilation, there are some other aspects we need to consider. We need to understand these to derive the maximum benefits from our tridoṣa profiles. In the following sections we will shift our focus to the principles that govern our ability to digest. Whatever we digest ultimately nourishes us and becomes us, and whatever we cannot will create problems for us.

Section Four

The Science of Digestion

The Process of Digestion
Causes of Indigestion
Aṣṭavidha Āhāra Vidhi Viśeṣāyatan
Dinacaryā: Daily Activities
Ṛtucaryā

The Science of Digestion

'You are what you eat . . .
No! You are what you digest!'

—Dr Sanjay Pisharodi

Some years ago, I was on holiday in Kuala Lumpur, Malaysia. I was looking forward to eating some good vegetarian Malaysian food, for how can a holiday be complete without good food? But to my dismay, when I landed in Kuala Lumpur, I did not feel hungry the entire week! The stomach was stubbornly uncooperative. My mood was disturbed too.

I wondered why it was so. I noticed that around noon, thundering clouds would appear in the sky and it would rain for a couple of hours. It would happen daily. I realized it was the weather that was killing my appetite. I, being from Mumbai, India, had a different biological set-up, which does not experience moist, cold weather at noon time. Hence, my appetite was lost. And then I tried to examine what people eat, especially the spices. I found they used a lot of ginger, sesame oil and soy sauce in their cuisines. All these are heat enhancers. Now, these are essential ingredients to raise the fire in the stomach for proper digestion. I realized I had to adapt to the local style of food whether I liked it or not.

The point is, you can't always just eat what you like, as the weather and other factors may not be conducive to that particular food. This becomes more obvious when we travel. I believe in the age-old saying—'Travelling makes a young man old'. As discussed earlier, nature designs our body for a certain climate, and when we travel we change our surroundings, but our body of course remains the same. So, there is a mismatch. Travelling is not something that can be avoided in today's age. So what does Ayurveda recommend? Generally, Ayurveda recommends that one eat local food. So, when I was in Malaysia, what I needed was to include more ginger or pepper or similar ingredients in my meals. We have discussed choosing the appropriate ingredients based on our prakṛti/nature and the role of spices in our digestion. But there is more to digestion.

The Process of Digestion

'A healthy outside begins from the inside.'

—Robert Urich

The most important factor in digestion is the digestive fire itself. If the digestive fire is strong, one can digest even iron nails. My grandfather and people from his generation, just to encourage us, used to say, 'When I was of your age I could digest rocks.' With the advent of the modern industrial era, the strength of car engines to burn fuel has gone up manifold, but the digestive fire in our stomachs has become weaker. Machines have taken away our physical labour and high-pressure jobs have increased our stress. Both have affected our digestive strength. The powerful warrior of mediaeval times used to digest large quantities of food. For example, the city palace museum of Udaipur lists the weight of weapons and armour of King Maharaja Rana Pratap at 35 kg or 75 pounds. Carrying this much weight on the body during battle required great strength, which was a result of the strength of digestion and pure food.

Let's turn our discussion to the process of digestion and the factors that govern our digestive fire. We can think of our digestive system as the hardware, over which we don't have a lot of control, as it is a function of our genetic makeup. But for it to run smoothly, we need to regulate our daily habits and also be mindful about adjusting our routine according to the season. The study of these habits is known as Dinacaryā and Ṛtucaryā, respectively, in Ayurveda. These habits are the software for our digestive system. If the software and hardware are in sync, everything will function smoothly. All the great Ayurvedic Ācāryas agree that it is better to prevent a disease condition than to keep treating it. Each of them speaks emphatically about the daily conduct for a healthy life. We will briefly discuss every aspect and connect it to the process of digestion.

Digestive System: The Hardware

Food primarily affects our body in six different ways. It nourishes (builds), reduces (emaciates), heats, cools, dries or moistens (oils) the body. So, we need to choose our diet depending on our requirements. For example, people who want to lose weight need to eat food that has the necessary effect. But results will show only if we are able to digest the food properly.

The process of digestion is akin to cooking itself. Ayurveda says that there is a constant fire in our stomach. It is similar to the flame of a stove burner, ignited when fuel is provided. In digestion, the pot is the stomach, the duodenum the stove, fuel the food that was digested earlier, and the digestive fire the flame. If the fire is too low, the food remains uncooked, and if the fire is too high, the food burns. It must be just right for digestion to take place smoothly.

The fact that we feel hungry is a sign of the presence of this fire. No hunger means no fire. Sometimes we may not feel hungry for days. That means the fire has been extinguished or is too low to arouse hunger. Overeating, cold humid weather, constipation, sleeplessness, insomnia and stress are some of the reasons for lack of hunger. Guided fasting helps the digestive fire or hunger to rise back.

The entire process of digestion is aided by kapha, vāta and pitta. Just as we need oil, water, air and fire to cook, during digestion, kapha supplies moisture and unctuousness, vāta supplies the air element as well as the movement of food and pitta supplies the fire to cook/digest. These active kapha, pitta and vāta are our body's secretions and reactions to the incoming food and independent of the kapha, pitta and vāta present in the food.

According to Ayurveda, the digestion process begins as soon as we see the food. The sight of food activates the system and releases various secretions. This begins in the mouth, where we have a type of kapha called bodhaka kapha ('bodhana' means 'to become aware'). The function of this kapha is to experience or become aware of the taste. The experience of the taste triggers the influence on other doṣas and the process of digestion proceeds. The food is then carried by vāta (prāṇa vāta) into the stomach. Another vāta (*samāna* vāta) holds the food in the stomach. This is known as samāna (which means stability/equilibrium) vāta. This vāta has the ability to retain the food for some time in the stomach to be digested. Next, another vāta known as *vyāna* vāta is activated in the small intestine or duodenum and is responsible for igniting the fire to start the actual digestion. The food to be cooked needs to be moistened and unctuous. This is done by another kapha in the upper part of the stomach (āmāśaya), known as *kledaka* kapha. Kledaka kapha moistens the food and makes it soft.

The word 'kledana' means 'to moisten'. Finally, the softened and moistened food particles are digested by pitta (*pācaka* pitta) which is the actual digestive fire. This is shown in Fig. 4.1 and Table 4.1. The pācaka pitta through proper digestion divides the food into two parts, essence (sāra) and waste (maḷa). When digestion is 100 per cent successful, we get only these two products, that is pure essence (sāra) and pure waste. The waste is pushed down with the help of another vāta called apāna vāta/vāyu into the large intestine and finally removed from the body through the anus.

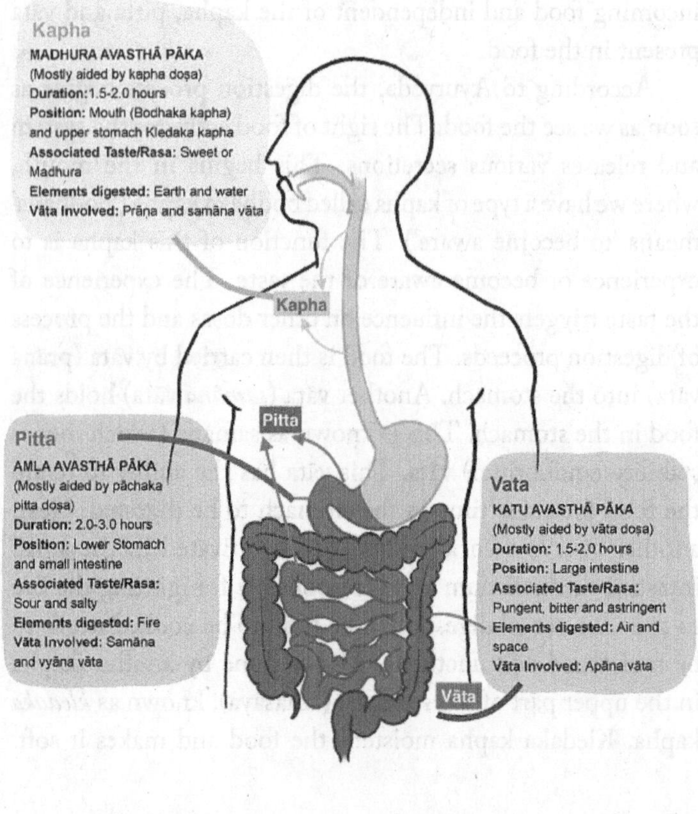

Although all three doṣas are active throughout the process of digestion, kapha is more active in the initial stage of digestion, pitta in the middle and vāta in the end (Table 4.1). When kapha is active, the rasa is sweet. It becomes sour during pitta phase and finally astringent during the vāta phase. The sāra or essence that is obtained as the main product of digestion is further processed and absorbed by the body.

Table 4.1: Process of Digestion

Active Doṣa	Location	Active Rasa	Digested elements	Duration
Kapha stage	Mouth to upper part of stomach	Sweet stage	Earth, Water	1.5—2 hours
Pitta stage	Lower part of stomach and small intestine	Sour stage	Fire	2—3 hours
Vāta stage	Colon and rectum	Pungent stage	Air, Ether	1.5—2 hours

Pitta is made up of fire and water elements. But what makes pācaka pitta (digestive fire) special is that the water element is practically absent, and it is a sharp fiery substance perfect for digesting or cooking the ingested food. This pācaka pitta is the foundational pitta in our body and supports all other pitta.

The digestion doesn't end at the production of essence (sāra) and waste (maḷa). The maḷa or waste is discarded, and the sāra is further processed. The sāra or essence produced by pācaka pitta is further digested by rañjaka pitta, to produce rakta dhātu or blood. Whatever is then left of the sāra is digested by various pitta in muscles, bones, marrow and semen to fortify these tissues. At every stage of digestion, a waste product accompanies the respective production. All the waste, apart from stool and urine (the waste product of primary digestion in stomach), manifests as dirt in eyes and ears, perspiration, nails and hair.

Improper pācaka pitta leads to indigestion, which means the fire is unable to completely transform food to sāra and waste, or the digestion is not 100 per cent. Then, apart from sāra (essence) and waste, a third by-product named āma (toxins) is produced in our stomach. The quantity of āma depends upon the extent of indigestion. This āma is the root cause of almost all diseases. And the same is true with all other digestive pitta(s) in various parts of the body. Wherever the digestive pitta fails to perform, toxins will be created along with tissue and waste, thus causing sickness.

These toxins may also block the smooth removal of waste products and thus cause more complications. All Ayurvedic texts thus contain principles and guidelines for perfect digestion, so that āma is not created, and people can lead a disease-free life. Thus, it is so essential to understand the causes of indigestion and take care of them.

Causes of Indigestion

Symptoms: When food is digested properly, any belch that is produced will be without smell or taste, and there won't be any pain in the abdomen or chest. Good digestion naturally creates a feeling of enthusiasm and happiness. It also provides a lot of energy and the waste (stool and urine) is ejected smoothly and regularly. The body feels light, and hunger and thirst recur naturally after a few hours.

Good digestion also keeps the tridoṣa in balance, brings clarity to the mind and maintains the life force. Indigestion, on the other hand, leads to many problems. The primary cause of indigestion is improper digestive fire. The undigested food in the stomach slowly ferments, causing one to burp over and again for a couple of hours or more after eating. Especially so if the stomach is unable to push the undigested food out. All these symptoms arise due to kapha imbalance. Vāta imbalance arising out of indigestion results in irregularities in nature's call and evacuation, weakness, body ache, headache, lower back pain and stiffness in the back. Pitta imbalance shows up as inability to taste, anorexia, burning sensation, thirst, ulcers in the mouth, acid reflux, nausea and gastritis. So, it is important to find out the causes of indigestion and address them well.

Generally, one needs to observe which doṣa is affected more and address it first (symptomatic treatment). For example, one needs to sip hot water if there is kapha- or vāta-related imbalance, and cool water in case of pitta imbalance. It is necessary to wait till the food has been ejected from the stomach before doing any light activity.

Causes: Disruption of digestive fire is of three types. When it is less intense, digestion doesn't take place. If it is too much, it burns the food, and if it is erratic it cooks partially. The causes, as you might have guessed, are due to imbalance in any of the doṣas. We saw how all the three doṣas are actively involved in digestion, and any imbalance would create disruption of digestive fire. The three disruptive digestive fires are *mandāgni* (weak fire) owing to excess kapha, *teekṣṇāgni* (intense fire) owing to excess pitta and *viṣamāgni* (erratic fire) owing to imbalance of vāta doṣa.

Mandāgni: Kapha, which is made up of earth and water, has the ability to extinguish digestive fire as both water and earth are anti-fire elements. When there is excess kapha in the stomach during digestion, it will naturally weaken the strength of digestive fire, resulting in mandāgni. This will slow down digestion and instead of seven to eight hours, it will take longer (Table 4.2). The result is production of āma. Āma is like a sticky watery substance we find in rotten food. This sticky fluid causes blockages in tissues and cells resulting in sluggish metabolism, blockages of toxins and excreta in the body, lowered immunity and poor nutrition. So, supply of fresh nutrients as well as removal of toxins gets blocked.

Restoring: The way to overcome this is to eat an anti-kapha diet. The diet should be light and easily digestible, and be prepared using more spices such as ginger, pepper, asafoetida, etc., and ingredients with less kapha, such as wheat, bottle gourd, fenugreek leaves, etc. Incorporating regular exercise and avoiding sleeping in the day also helps overcome this problem. In this way, once the light food starts getting digested, the fire will steadily gain strength, and be restored through exercises and yoga āsanas. *Agnisāra kriyā*, a yoga regime, along with nauli (a type of exercise) restores jatharāgni or digestive fire. The word Agnisāra is a composite of two words—'agni' which means 'fire' and 'sāra' which means 'essence'. So, this kriyā or activity restores the digestive fire and prevents kapha from affecting the digestion.

The agnisāra kriyā is done as follows:

1. Stand on your yoga mat with the feet about 12–16 inches apart.
2. Slightly bend the knees.
3. Place your palms on your knees while slightly bending forward. Keep your spine straight and at 45 degrees to the floor.
4. Exhale slowly and completely (as you bend down to place your palms on your knees), eliminating all the air from the lungs.
5. Suck the core abdominal muscles in, pulling the navel back toward the spine.
6. Lower the chin to the chest and lock the throat.
7. Now, without breathing, relax the muscles of the abdomen and start moving these muscles in and out at rapidly. Try to maintain a smooth movement. Do it till you can hold your breath.

8. Inhaling slowly, return to the standing position.

Repeat instructions 1–8 five times. Do this on an empty stomach, preferably early in the morning. Nauli kriyā is an advanced version of agnisāra kriyā, where the abdominal muscle is rotated in circular movement. This greatly helps to increase digestive fire.

It's also possible that the pācaka pitta is low when there is excess water. As a result, digestion slows down and takes longer. This is similar to mandāgni though the kapha is in balance. The remedial measure is similar to mandāgni.

Teekṣṇāgni: Excess pitta causes intense fire, leading to quick digestion. In this case, the digestive fire burns the food instead of digesting it, whether the food is raw or cooked. The person with Teekṣṇāgni may feel satisfied momentarily but will soon become restless and hungry. The sāra or essence, which is the nourishing nutritional juice (to be carried to different parts of the body), does not form due to excess heat and dryness. One also feels frequent hunger and thirst, and even after eating multiple times one does not feel satisfaction as the body fails to get nutrition. This happens when the water element in pāchaka pitta reduces almost to zero. The excess heat also reduces kapha and its activity to build the body. So, tissues deplete and high heat pitta along with vāta destroy the body.

Restoration: The immediate remedy is consumption of a pitta-balancing diet. Charaka advises curbing the fire by supplying heavy food (high kapha and calorie) in large quantities to curb the fire. This should be supplied again and again. The body will regain nutrition and the tridoṣa will gain balance. Over a period of time, the digestive fire will normalize. Heavy exercise is not recommended for this condition. Staying awake late at night will only exacerbate the symptoms.

Viṣamāgni: Erratic or irregular digestive fire is most difficult to control. Of all the three doṣas, delocalized subtle vāta is difficult to control, so when the disruption in digestive fire is due to vāta imbalance, the situation is viṣam, which literally means dangerous. Vāta can make the fire strength increase or decrease, or let it stay just right. Samāna vāta, which controls the digestive fire in the small intestine at the point of connection with the stomach is very crucial. The name samāna means 'balanced on both sides'. That means when pāchaka pitta is too high, samāna vāta should be reduced, and when it is low, the samāna vāta should gradually increase to raise the strength of fire. But when samāna vāta itself goes out of control, the situation is viṣam or unpredictably dangerous. When the samāna vāta is too high it will result in teekṣṇāgni (high) and when low it will make digestive fire slow down, or mandāgni.

Restoration: The remedy is a vāta balancing diet that focuses on spices such as ginger, asafoetida and pepper. Heavy food (cheese, paneer, chickpeas, etc.) should be avoided and simple rice, moong dal soup and fresh wholewheat bread with a good quantity of ghee is good for the body. Great millet (jawāri) rotis with ghee are also recommended. Since an imbalanced vāta quickly throws pitta and kapha out of balance, one should be vigilant and simultaneously address those imbalances.

Samāgni: When all the three doṣas are in balance and contribute cooperatively, digestion is smooth and at an optimum level.

However, apart from tridoṣa, the process of digestion depends on many other factors. For example, if we eat the right food but at the wrong time, then we will not be able to digest it. So, we will next discuss various important rules that need to be followed for complete digestion.

Asṭavidha Āhāra Vidhi Viśeṣāyatan

'We think we eat Anna or food, but in reality Anna eats us!'

—Ayurvedic proverb

We saw how a perfect Ayurvedic meal is that which is easily digested, provides nourishment to all tissues, does not create toxins (āma) and does not create imbalance in the tridoṣa. How do we achieve this? Earlier, whenever people would talk about food, they would naturally think of its attributes, such as kapha, pitta, vāta, heavy and light, strength of digestive fire, etc. It was an integral part of their lives and cooking. But nowadays, we only speak of how yummy the food is. However, the Ayurvedic principles are not rocket science. The more we use these concepts in our diet, the more accustomed to them we will become. No one knows your body and digestion better than yourself. Being able to discern what you need and what you should eat will take you closer to good health.

Ayurveda recommends eightfold rules for proper digestion of food. This is known as *Asṭavidha Āhāra Vidhi Viśeṣāyatan*. Practising these rules make us aquatinted with Ayurvedic lifestyle and proper digestion. These eight golden rules are as follows:

1. ***prakṛti*** or the nature of the food
2. ***karana*** or proper cooking or preparation of food
3. ***saṃyoga*** or a proper menu of items/preparations
4. ***rāshi*** or appropriate quantity
5. ***deśa*** or geographical region
6. ***kāla*** or time of eating (day as well as season)
7. ***upayoga-samstha*** or appropriate hunger level
8. ***upabhokta*** or the consumer of the food

When we take care of all the above eight factors, we will be able to digest the food. If any one is neglected, digestion will be hampered to the extent that the rule is overlooked. What if we do not digest the food? The undigested food will degenerate into unhygienic toxins (āma), disturb the balance of the doṣas and start shaking the very foundation of our life. In other words, the food we don't digest starts eating us away. Ayurveda boldly says that all diseases take birth in our stomach. Let's have a closer understanding of these eight aspects of food consumption, which are integral for a long, disease-free life.

1. **Prakṛti (Qualities)**: Apart from doṣa constitution of ingredients, dravya guṇa (not triguṇa) or food qualities affect digestion. We have discussed these qualities in Section Two which are: six tastes and qualities that include whether an ingredient is heavy/light, dry/moist, sharp/gross, what vīrya or potency (hot/cold) it possesses and its vipāka or taste after digestion. The state of our digestive fire also allows us to understand what food we should eat. For example, when our digestive fire is high, we can eat heavy food such as cheese. Milk, which is lighter but has similar nourishing ability, can

be consumed when the digestive fire is normal. When the fire is weak, we should have buttermilk with ginger.

As we've discussed earlier, food with hot potency is good for kapha prakṛti people (or when our kapha is high), whereas food with cooling potency is good for persons with pitta prakṛti (or when our pitta is high). Madhura rasa or sweet taste nourishes kapha prakṛti, whereas pungent ignites pitta and bitter aggravates vāta doṣa. The last is vipāka or the 'after-effects'. What rasa the food becomes after digestion will affect the doṣas accordingly. If it is sweet, it will balance pitta and if pungent it will increase the pitta doṣa.

2. **Karana:** This refers to the processing and cooking of the ingredients. The purpose of cooking is to transform something that is indigestible so that it is easily digested. This transformation is called samskāra which literally means activities that purify the food to a superior state. For example, rice is heavy in its raw unclean stage. The simple samskāra of washing the grains with water makes it light. And passing it through Agni samskāra or cooking with fire makes it even lighter. So, the cook should always remember that the whole focus of cooking is to purify the food so that one can digest it easily.

Good, clean food is tempting and fragrant, and the very sight and smell of it stimulates the digestive system.

Another example of a food that needs to be adapted to the situation is yoghurt. Yoghurt in itself is heavy and disturbs pitta doṣa. But when it is diluted with water and undergoes the samskāra of churning, the resultant buttermilk is not only light to digest but also mitigates the disturbed pitta doṣa.

Similarly, heavy legumes, such as black gram (urad dal), can be rendered light by soaking in water for seven to eight hours. There are so many such processes—many that we have discussed in the section on different ingredients—that a cook should practise to make the food digestible. Apart from cleaning, cooking on fire and churning, samskāra includes adding natural flavouring and preserving agents, storing food in appropriate pots and serving them in the right dish. We should not store or serve, for example, sour food in copper and silver pots. All this when done properly, enhances the experience of and pleasure of eating manifold.

3. Saṃyoga and Viruddha Āhāra: The choice of menu or the combination of different preparations served for consumption should be chosen to create synergy. Synchronized combinations of food are called saṃyoga or compatible (sama means equal and yoga means connection). When the combinations are incompatible, it falls under Viruddha Āhāra. Viruddha means opposing or contradicting. Ācārya Vāgabhaṭa classifies Viruddha Āhāra under poisoned foods, because the wrong combinations create toxins, infect blood, destroy tissues and become a potential source of diseases. Sometimes two items with opposing qualities may create indigestion while sometimes even a combination of two similar items may create similar problems. Two items with opposing qualities may nullify each others' positive impacts, whereas two similar items may sum up and amplify each other's negative qualities to the point of poisonous effect. Some of these are bloating, vomiting, diarrhoea and skin allergies. Ayurveda enumerates many different reasons that lead to Viruddha Āhāra. Some of them are: saṃyoga or a proper menu of items/preparations.

Deśa (Place) Viruddha: Eating very dry food or drinking strong wine in a dry climate will lead to a dangerous increase in vāta and pitta doṣas. Similarly, oily and cold food should be avoided completely in marshy areas. Places like Dubai, which have a dry climate due to proximity to the desert, may have air-conditioning in all buildings and cars but these are just artificial barriers that protect us temporarily.

Kāla (Time) Viruddha: Eating cold and dry food in winter results in an increase in vāta and kapha doṣa. Extremely pungent/hot food in summer will disturb pitta. These are examples of diets that contradict the characteristics of the time when they are consumed.

Agni (Digestive Fire/Abilities) Viruddha: Eating heavy food when the digestive fire is low (mandāgni) or eating light food when the digestive fire is high (teekshṇāgni) falls under digestive fire contradictions.

Mātrā **(Dose) Viruddha:** An imbalance can occur when two ingredients are combined in the wrong proportion. It is not healthy to consume yoghurt with an equal amount of honey.

Sātmya Viruddha: Sātmya here refers to the way a child is brought up in his/her food habits. A person accustomed to pungent and hot food will experience indigestion if they eat a lot of food that is sweet and cold.

Prakṛti Viruddha: Diet that is prakṛti-friendly but against the sātmya falls under this category. Sātmya can develop opposed to prakṛti due to persistent bad habits.

Samskāra (Process/Cooking) Viruddha: This refers to cooking procedures that make the ingredient unfit for consumption. For example, honey can be added to hot water but should not be heated directly.

Vīrya (Potency) Viruddha: Combining food with contradictory potency like fish (hot) with milk (cold) can be a cause of indigestion. This applies in a few cases and not every cold–hot potency combination is contradictory.

***Kostha* (Bowel) Viruddha:** This condition arises when a person needs to take special care of their diet or when to eat because of the condition of their bowels. For example, a person whose bowels are soft should not be given any heavy food and vice-versa.

***Avasthā* (Situation) Viruddha:** When the food does not suit the condition, it can lead to indigestion. For example, eating vāta-aggravating food after a spell of hard physical labour, exercise or sexual intercourse, or having kapha-dominant cold food after a long spell of sleep.

***Krama* (Sequence) Viruddha:** Eating before clearing the bowel or urinary bladder will cause issues. Drinking milk after curd rice will increase kapha doṣa.

***Pāka* (Cooking) Viruddha:** Using a bad fuel for cooking, undercooking, overcooking or burning the food causes indigestion.

Saṃyoga (Combination) Viruddha: As discussed, indigestion is caused when two ingredients don't combine well. For example, sour food with milk.

Hṛdaya **(Liking) Viruddha:** If the food we eat is unpalatable or unappealing to us, we will be unable to digest it. So, healthy food needs to be tasty too. However, taste buds vary from person to person. I know people who do not like the taste of ghee. So, they can't digest ghee although it is one of the healthiest foods.

Vidhi **(Procedure) Viruddha:** Eating in the right environment, such as in a quiet, comfortable place in the company of family and friends is far more conducive to proper digestion than eating in a noisy, unfamiliar place.

At this point, you're probably wondering, 'But how do I determine which food would suit *me* and what should *I* avoid?' The best rule is to stick to simple, unadulterated food that you have loved since childhood and that hasn't made you fall ill. Now, with more and more food of different cuisines available to us easily, it's possible for the system to get confused and for us to fall sick.

It's good to sample new food and recipes once in a while but stick to familiar food you find delicious for most meals. While exploring new cuisines, be mindful of what is conducive, how much it resembles your usual diet and what might be tough for the system to take in. If something new, no matter how tasty, makes you uncomfortable, make sure you don't repeat the mistake of eating it again. Apart from this, there are certain combinations that are universally bad. These are summarized in Table 4.2.

Table 4.2: Examples of Incompatible Foods

Item	Incompatible with
Milk	Sour fruits, excess salt, sprouted grains, garlic, radish, moringa, holy basil, yoghurt, cheese,
Spinach	Sesame seeds
Honey	Equal quantity of ghee or water, sesame oil, sugar
Radish	Black gram
Curds	Palm dates
Banana	Buttermilk
Sprouts	Lotus stems

4. Rāshi/Quantity: Once you are sure about the quality of the food, and the right combinations for your body, you must focus on the quantity of food to be eaten. The simplest way to determine this is eating according to how hungry you are. But never confuse hunger and craving. Craving is an intense hankering triggered by the mind and not from the stomach. On the other hand, real hunger rises from the abdomen. A typical craving draws us to some tasty confectionery or savoury food. We can satisfy hunger but not the craving, because hunger is a natural urge. But craving falls in the category of greed. Cravings are what cause us to overeat. In fact, the very first bite may be an act of overeating. Cravings tend to arise at stressful moments, when we are bored or trying to distract ourselves. So, we must distinguish between hunger and craving. Natural hunger will make us want food, but not be too picky and gratefully accept whatever is served. Of course, you must still be vigilant that the food will suit you.

Ayurveda recommends that we should eat according to the strength of our digestive fire. If the fire is weak, then eat less and if it is more, eat more. If we eat more in the case of a weak fire, and less in case of more, we will fall sick.

Some diet plans encourage people to eat less than they need to, which is not good for overall health as the digestive secretions will start eating up the organs and affect how they function. The tissues in the body will be deprived of proper nourishment. Such dieting is based more on the mind's goal to achieve something, such as weight loss, while misusing the digestive system. The same happens when we neglect hunger in our passion to achieve something. Deadlines are good, but we should not be wrung out by the time we reach our goal.

Vāgabhaṭa says one should avoid eating till they are stuffed. Rather, eat only half of any heavy food (wheat, dairy, black gram, etc.) that you set out to. For example, if you feel like eating a full pizza, eat half instead. And supplement the gap with light food (say a salad) by three-fourths of one's estimate. Never stuff yourself 100 per cent. This is also overeating. A proper quantity of food is that which we are able to comfortably digest without feeling overwhelmingly hungry.

But how do you know if your hunger is satisfied? This is observed more so when the digestive fire is proper. In case of very low or high fire it will be difficult to notice this and the burps in such situation will carry the smell or taste of undigested food. Hence we need to be more mindful while eating. Also, when we eat the right amount, we digest the food in four to five hours and feel light. That is confirmation that we have eaten the right quantity.

Ayurveda says that some categories of food need to be eaten more than others. For example, we are not supposed to satiate our hunger only with deep fried snacks or just the food we love to eat. Taste and combinations need to be balanced too. There should be fewer bitter items than sour, and fewer sour items than sweet. Here, sweet does not mean confectionary, rather grains that have a natural sweet taste, such as rice and wheat flour. If need be, a small confectionary can be eaten at the beginning of the meal to stimulate interest and ignite the fire.

The sequence of eating should be from heavy to light food. Because when the fire is strong, heavy food can be digested well. We should then proceed to eat lighter food. In some traditions, sweets are offered at the end of the meal. Sweet taste imparts satisfaction to the mind and prevents one from overeating other food items. Once we have received the sweet, it is customary to say to the server, 'Thank you. I am satisfied and no more food please.'

5. Deśa/Place: We briefly discussed the place of eating in the Viruddha Āhāra section. Certain food should not be eaten at certain places. But perhaps even more important is knowing where the ingredient is coming from. Where is it cultivated and in what manner? In a metropolis, one typically goes to the supermarket to buy ingredients. It is difficult to determine the finer details of the origin of the ingredients.

Ayurveda divides places into three categories: desert, marshy land and places with moderate climate. Deserts are dry regions, which could be due to heat or cold. The food that grows in such areas has more vāta doṣa due to prevalent dryness in the climate. For example, eggplants from a dry climate will have more vāta than those growing in marshy areas where it is humid, and the result is increased kapha doṣa. People who grew up in a dry climate will find the food from the same area more conducive as the food will be sātmya (united as one with their body). So when we migrate or travel from a place with one type of climate to another, we need to keep this in mind and gradually try to develop the necessary sātmya.

6. Kāla/Time: Time moves in periodic cycles and every cycle pushes us towards old age. However, the influence of time can be slowed if we know how to live with it. Eating at the right time is considered to be of the utmost importance. Those who eat at a fixed time in response to hunger enjoy the best of health. Those who eat according to the response of hunger and after digesting the previous meal relish good health too. Feeling hungry every day at the same time and being able to clear the bowels completely every morning is a blessing that everyone should aim for.

Ayurveda speaks of two types of time cycles. The first is nityag kāla, which refers to daily as well as seasonal cycles. Nityag means the eternal time cycle, repeating over and over again. One should have two meals a day for best health and avoid eating at night as the digestive fire is low. At night, one should rest the body as well as the digestive system. Similarly, due to the cold in winter, the digestive fire gets trapped and hunger rises considerably in a strong healthy body. At such time, heavy food in higher quantities is recommended. During summer, cool drinks and moist food are recommended. In the rainy season, when the digestive fire is very weak, one should cut down on eating as well as recreational activities. Sādhus or saintly people in India used to stay at one place for the four months of downpour and perform various austerities. We should also note that special care needs to be taken during the transition of seasons. We will discuss more on this in Ṛtucaryā later in this section.

The second type of time cycle is called 'avasthika kāla' which refers to three stages of life-span, *bālya* or childhood, *yauvana* or youth and *vṛdhya* or old age. This time structure, though appearing linear, is actually cyclic, to those who understand how we live in many life cycles. Like the silkworm who becomes a butterfly, the soul never dies. The silkworm experiences two life cycles. Death is just a passing phase when we change bodies. This is a sobering thought while examining death, especially untimely deaths. However, while living in a particular body, one has the *adhikār* or right to live a healthy life. During childhood, kapha is high; pitta is high during youth and vāta during old age. One needs to eat food with the opposite nature to balance the excess doṣa accumulations during a particular avastha of time span. During youth, one should be vigilant about spikes in pitta doṣa by eating cooling food (not chilled deserts or ice creams, but food that is cool in potency, like mint or cucumber). Likewise, one needs to avoid food with high vāta during the third phase of life.

Food with high kapha doṣa should be regulated in childhood. It's important to remember that a child also needs heavy kapha food to be able to grow strong, but it is important not to overeat. Similarly, a young person needs stimulation from pitta doṣa to think, act and grow, and older people need vāta to move. So, one needs to achieve a fine balance. Exercising and doing yoga helps maintain the balance throughout all the three phases of life.

7. Upayoga Samsthā or Mindful Eating: The foundational rule in this section is that the previous meal should be completely digested before ingesting new food. Complete digestion of the previous meal is usually signalled by clean belches or burps, enthusiasm to eat, feeling light in the body and proper manifestation of hunger and thirst. Prior to this, there is smooth evacuation of urges (like passing of stool and urine).

A healthy person, after making sure that they are feeling well, should eat wholesome food that is hot and freshly cooked, in proper quantity and not comprised of incompatible combinations, not too fast or too slow, in a proper place and with the right utensils, with full concentration, without talking or laughing.

8. Upabhoktā or the Consumer: Before consuming the food, one should also consider their situation. You should always communicate with the cook about your sātmya food habits, digestive fire, etc. Ultimately, this sincerity brings you the desired health through food. One should follow the rules as part of self-care.

Now you may feel it is very tough to follow all these rules in this modern day and time where life is so demanding and moves swiftly. There will be some breaks and our digestive fire may get affected. So, we will discuss how to restore digestive fire or improve it through yoga and certain rituals and habits that should be adopted during the day, night and various seasons.

Improving Digestion through Yoga

Yoga aligns our body, senses and mind with the supreme will, which is *'sarve sukhinām bhavantu'*—let everyone be happy.

These activities include yogic kriyās, āsana, prāṇāyāma, *prtyāhāra*, *dhāraṇā*, *dhyāna* and *samādhī*. We will discuss those which are exclusively helpful to improve digestion. Fasting also helps improve digestive fire. We will start with kriyās.

Kriyās: Agnisāra kriyā is very effective at improving digestive fire strength. This is especially useful for those with mandāgni. Do this five times early in the morning or when the stomach is empty. The advanced version of this is called 'nauli', which needs to be done under guidance.

Other kriyās include emesis, which involves drinking a lot of water, almost till the point of discomfort. This is very effective in removing kapha and pitta imbalance and correcting digestive fire. This is especially effective for teekṣṇāgni.

Another method to improve digestive fire is *vasti* kriyā or enema, wherein clean warm water is injected through the rectum to clean the long intestine. This balances disturbed vāta and is effective at overcoming viṣamāgni or erratic digestive fire. Ayurveda says that vasti is half of all the treatments put together. These kriyās are standard yogic practices and there is nothing to feel embarrassed about. My father-in-law, who is seventy-four years old and regularly does enema, is very healthy and is as energetic as if he is in his fifties. He is strict about his diet too.

Kriyās are meant for all adults as well, and if done from a young age, one will enjoy a healthy body throughout their life. Just as we clean our mouth by brushing, we must clean other orifices too. For years and decades, day in and day out we keep sending food down our alimentary canal. At times, it needs to be cleaned. These kriyās are basically cleansing processes that restore all the three doṣas in the digestive system to equilibrium.

One can do enema for three consecutive days and only once in twenty-four hours. We should specifically go for enema/vasti when the vāta doṣa increases. It will also effectively reduce our back pain and sciatica pain. I try doing it once a week, while followers of naturopathy recommend you do it every day. In case of doubt, consult Ayurvedic doctors and yoga teachers. Vasti/enema should not be practised by anyone with high blood pressure, hernia or any serious digestive disorders.

Post these kriyās, one needs to rest and restart the digestive system slowly. Initially, one should eat very light, semi-liquid food (such as soups) with a good quantity of ghee and little or no spices. Once the hunger returns, one can start eating normally.

Kriyās cleanse our body and improve digestion. Yoga āsanas then strengthen the digestive organs and makes them robust, and prāṇāyāma strengthens our mental faculties. The *ardha-matsendriya* āsana (spinal twist), *pavana mukta* āsana (removing air from intestines), sarvānga āsana (shoulder stand posture) and halāsana (plough pose) are very useful in restoring digestive fire. These āsanas should be done under guidance. I learnt yoga lessons in Sivananda Yoga Vidya Peetham in Uttarkashi, which is situated at the foothills of the Himalayas and next to the holy river Gangā, under the guidance of Swami Govindananda Saraswati. Another place that teaches authentic yoga is Anand Prakash Yoga Ashram (Rishikesh, India) of Yogrishi Vishvketu. I myself teach a few students in the morning every day. Any yoga teacher trained from such places can help you practise these āsanas, prāṇāyāma and kriyās.

Prāṇāyāma and dhyāna or meditation, will help to regulate our mind's activities and thus better handle residual stresses.

Air is the subtlest among the five gross elements that build our body, and is the connection between body and mind. So, by regulating one's breathing, one can increase the strength of one's mind. Proper breathing techniques are effective exercise for the mind as much as weightlifting is exercise for the arm muscles. Prāṇāyāma is effective in keeping the digestive system working properly with increasing age. As we age, mental stress increases, so we need to increase these activities with time. The amount of time on physical āsanas will reduce proportionally as we increase the time spent on prāṇāyāma and meditation. Meditation works from within and is more effective in increasing mental strength than prāṇāyāma. However, meditation is possible only after regulating one's mind through prāṇāyāma. Both prāṇāyāma and meditation require rigorous guidance from experienced yoga teachers.

Improving Digestion through Fasting

Fasting is also a part of the Yoga regime and helps improve digestive fire. Fasting rekindles our hunger and digestive fire. Fasting is basically allowing the digestive system to rest. All the accumulated toxins are removed from the alimentary canal. All the three doṣas get balanced and gradually the hunger arises with a healthy digestive fire.

When should one fast? Usually, the eleventh lunar day is the best day to fast, as on a full moon night as well as on a dark moon night, the water element in our body goes through a lot of agitation. Just as the moon affects oceans, it affects the water in our body too. So, fasting on the eleventh lunar day (called Ekādaśi) helps one handle the influence better. One should begin preparing for the fasting a day before. On the tenth lunar day, one should eat light and have a simple soup as dinner. On the eleventh day, one should not eat grains and cooked food, but only sweet fruits. One should also avoid strenuous physical and mental activities. The day and night should be passed reflecting and meditating on the higher purpose of life. On such days, we need to keep the mind absorbed on higher purposes rather than material and bodily desires, or it will create anxiety and defeat the purpose of fasting.

On the following day, on Dwadashi, one should break the fast with lemon juice or even better, with fresh gooseberry juice mixed with warm water and a pinch of salt. This helps cleanse the intestine thoroughly. Then, after clearing the bowels and bathing, one can start the day with light food. The food will feed the digestive fire and in due course, one will get proper hunger and return to a normal diet.

There are two more basic aspects of yoga. They are *yama* and *niyama* or rules and regulations for healthy life. These rules and regulations make one eligible to practise āsana, prāṇāyāma and so on. In Ayurveda, such rules and regulations are described as Dinacaryā and Ṛtucaryā.

Dinacaryā: Daily Activities

'Never go to sleep without a request to your sub-consciousness.'

—Thomas Edison

A successful day begins the previous night. Life becomes wonderful when we take it one day a time, and consistently find peace, happiness and stability. And after years, when we look back, our hearts will be filled with satisfaction. Ayurveda, although it treats and cures all types of sicknesses, trains one in a lifestyle that would prevent one from falling sick. Daily routines are a very powerful means to keep one safe and secure from a variety of health issues.

Night Regime: Of all the night regimes, sleep is the most important. A good sound rest can help abate half of the afflictions we experience. Most of us have seen how sleep can soothe a throbbing headache and even bring down a fever. If our meals are properly digested, our mind is free from stress and pitta is calm during sleep, we can look forward to a very robust and energetic day.

For good rest, dinner should be chosen very carefully. An early, light dinner leads to a good night's sleep. Eating at night should be done before or after the sun sets. Earlier, we discussed how morning hours are kapha, noon is pitta and afternoon till sunset is vāta. During the evening, while the sun is setting and when the doṣas are in transition, it is better not to eat. According to Vāgabhaṭa, one can have a light dinner during the first three hours of the night, i.e. between 6 and 9 p.m. And because that is kapha hour, and digestive fire is low, it is better to eat light. After dinner, one should wash hands, mouth and feet, brush teeth, and wash the eyes with fresh cooling water. All these activities are meant to balance excess pitta. Light walking helps to digest the dinner while the fresh air of moonlit night calms pitta and increases sexual desire.

The suppression of sexual desire leads to a lot of health issues. One should avoid sex during the mornings, sunset, mid-day and midnight. The best time for sex is during the end of the kapha hours of the evening (8–10 p.m.). After sex, to revitalize, one is advised to take a shower, bask in cool breeze and drink milk with sugar. One should retire to sleep before commencement of pitta hours. 7–10 p.m. is predominated by kapha prakṛti. After that period, pitta becomes prominent and then vāta. So, if there is indigestion, it will disturb our sleep during pitta hours as pitta will have to work to digest the remaining food. Because of this, the quality of sleep will be hampered and despite spending seven to eight hours in bed, we will wake up tired. That will potentially ruin our day. Those having excess pitta are recommended to have triphalā curṇa with ghee before sleeping. Also washing the feet and face calms pitta and helps one rest better. A foot massage with oil and a light dry massage also helps one sleep better.

The cooler the body is during sleep, the better will be the quality of rest and not hampered by dreams. This is possible if the heating system of our body, that is the digestive system, is resting before the body rests. It is also important that the mind is calm. Watching horror movies or checking stock prices just before sleeping is not a good idea. We should switch off all background processes before calling it a day.

Yoga nidrā or being connected with sleep means to be away from our body, mind and senses for a while. It is the art of withdrawing oneself from the surroundings, which in turn encourages relaxation and sleep. Although the original purpose of yoga nidrā is to be connected with the supreme bliss which lies beyond body and senses, a good sleep is a natural side-effect in the first place. Many of my students slip off to sleep during a yoga nidrā session.

Day Regime: Ayurveda recommends rising during Brahma Muhurta, roughly one and half hours before sunrise. In countries closer to the north or south poles, this will need adjustment, but the basic principle is to rise after seven hours of rest while it is still dark. During Brahma Muhurta, all the three doṣas of nature are balanced. Rising at this time and in this state allows one to experience a serene peace that is unmatched by the rest of the day.

Evacuating: Centuries ago, people would eat at home and then step out of the house to respond to the urges of the bowels and bladder. Hence the term 'Nature's call'. But now there is no reason to step out of home. It has increased convenience but has done away with the short morning walk that effectively prepares one to clear one's bowels completely. When the bowel clears, the accumulated vāta, especially from the last hours of sleep, is also removed from the body. If the vāta is not cleared, it affects the digestive fire adversely, and the entire day's regime can get affected.

Mouth Cleansing: After clearing the bowels, one should brush one's teeth with a natural bitter/astringent tree twigs. This should be done without hurting the gums. Astringent is a very good cleansing agent, whereas the bitter neem twigs disinfects the mouth completely. It also balances the kapha and pitta within the mouth. Sweet twigs balance pitta and vāta. In general, cleansing the mouth removes accumulated kapha doṣa and strengthens the gums. One should scrape the tongue using a scraper made from either gold, silver or stainless steel. A deep cleanse mouth washing includes oil pulling (different oil is used for different prakṛti, but sesame oil is good for all prakṛti).

Oil pulling should be done before brushing. It is very useful in keeping the teeth strong and removing toxins. All you need to do is take a teaspoon of oil and hold it in the mouth for as long as you can (maximum five minutes). Keep swishing the oil slowly within your mouth. Then spit it out and rinse your mouth with water. The mouth is the gateway to the alimentary canal, and it needs to be clean to receive the food that is prepared with so much care. If it is clean, the taste buds on the tongue respond well and release all the required secretions in the mouth, so that chewing and mixing can take place smoothly. Digestion of carbohydrates begins in the mouth. The saliva secreted from your salivary glands moistens food as it's chewed. Saliva releases an enzyme called amylase, which begins the breakdown process of the sugars in the carbohydrates you're eating. So, proper chewing and secretion is important. The proteins are mostly digested by enzymes secreted in the stomach. Thus, it is important to chew your food more when you are eating vegetarian food. Ayurveda says we should chew thirty-two times or till the solid food almost turns into liquid before it passes to the stomach. Even among animals, you'll notice that herbivores chew for a long time before swallowing. On the other hand, carnivores just tear and swallow meat. We are omnivores, so we need to cook vegetables (as well as meat) and chew properly for digestion. For all this to happen effectively, we need to make sure our mouth is clean. Similarly, after eating, we need to clean the mouth, hands and feet to enhance digestion.

Massaging: Ayurveda recommends massaging the body with oil before bathing. Oil massage balances vāta, makes the skin shiny and healthier, and improves sense perception. A foot massage removes fatigue and improves vision by pacifying vāta and a pitta doṣa called *alochaka*. Vāgabhaṭa says that the important areas of massage are the head, ears and feet. Massaging ends with adding tiny drops of warm oil to the nose. This is called nāsyam and should be done daily. Initially, this may be done under supervision with someone's help. Nāsyam is very helpful for the health of the neck and senses grouping around the nose, eyes and ears. The nose is the gateway to the head, and taking care of it is essential.

Exercises: Many years ago, when I was in the prime of my youth and health, I got a chance to go to Badrinath in the Himalayas. There, on the third day, we trekked for seven to eight kilometres on snow-clad mountainous terrains to visit Vasudhārā, a beautiful, auspicious waterfall surrounded by glaciers. After spending an hour or so, we had to hurry back to our camp. The trek took up the entire day. That night, I experienced nausea and fever. I couldn't eat much, though a feast was laid out for us. I could feel the impact of that arduous exercise manifesting as fever.

Vāgabhaṭa advises that one should exercise according to one's capacity. A very healthy and strong person should use only half their capacity to exercise. And others should do even less. Too much exercise, according to Vāgabhaṭa, causes nausea, thirst, bleeding, debility (without working), headache and even fever. When I read that, I could easily relate it to my experience. I also recall a couple of other persons in the camp getting mild fever the same night. Too much exercise also leads to excess weight loss. While it is important to keep unhealthy weight gain in check, working out too much and eating too little is the wrong way to keep it in check. Rather, one should gradually reduce weight and remain healthy while doing so. The whole purpose of exercise is to gain strength, not to lose it. A good, balanced exercise removes aggravations of the kapha and vāta doṣas and strengthens digestive fire. It makes one eager to eat good food and be able to digest it too. A kapha prakṛti person may exercise till they sweat well, a pitta person till some beads of perspiration appear on the forehead and a vāta person should do just joint movements. One should also not exercise in sickness and while experiencing indigestion. Exercise/yoga āsanas opens up the skin and the massaged oil nourishes the skin tissues.

Bathing: After exercise, one needs to relax for a few minutes before bathing. Bathing cleanses the body, brings vigour and ignites the digestive fire. Bathing with cool water pacifies pitta. In case of aggravated kapha and vāta, one should bathe with warm/hot water. The head should not be washed with hot water unless there are severe kapha and vāta imbalances.

After bathing, it is a custom to offer prayers to the gods and one's forefathers before starting the day. One can also perform prāṇāyāma and chant various mantras (like Oṁ) for preparing the mind to face the day.

All these activities cleanse the body as well as the mind. They are extremely useful in keeping a digestive system healthy. Classified as nitya karma or daily duties, an average person would spend nearly two hours on this regime. Now this seems difficult in a modern day setup, but we can always plan and find ways to apply the same principles. Earlier, physical exercise was an integral part of a person's daily activities. Now, we have to plan it separately as our work most often does not include heavy physical labour. Whether you choose walking, jogging, yoga, sports or gymming, some sort of exercise for an hour must feature in a daily schedule. Otherwise, it will affect your digestion and lead to various health issues.

After bathing, one should wear clean fresh clothes. Clothes should be woven from natural linen, cotton, silk, leather or wool, and worn according to the weather. It is considered that white clothes pacify pitta and vāta, and red pacifies kapha. Thin, soft clothing balances all the doṣas and increases appetite.

All the above regulated activities keep the digestive fire at its optimum level. Now, let's examine how the diet should be regulated.

Diet during a Typical Day

The morning hours, till 9 a.m., are dominated by kapha prakṛti. During this time, our digestive fire is not too high.

So we should eat easily digestible food. Soaked dried fruits and nuts are a good option. They are full of vitamins, essential fat, oils and minerals. Soaking them overnight cools the potency, making them easier to digest and helps to balance one's accumulated pitta from the previous night. If one still feels hungry, fruits or cooked food such as oats and pohā, which are easy to digest, are good options.

As the day progresses, hunger arises. The influence of pitta begins around 9.30–10 a.m., and the stomach responds to it. If someone is physically active from the morning, they could feel hungry enough as early as 10 a.m. and accordingly consume a freshly cooked hot square meal. If the lifestyle is sedentary, the hunger may come as late as 2 p.m. (this could also be the case if the breakfast hasn't been digested well). But it's important to wait to eat till one is hungry. It is best if lunch is eaten before or around noon.

Then one can have a snack around 4 or 5 p.m. as the vāta phase begins. Usually, we are drawn towards fried foods such as hot samosas or pakoras during this time, which has enough oil to balance the rising vāta. Of course, one should not eat fried food every day and in all seasons. But if one has to eat, this is the right time, only if you don't have a vāta imbalance or any other health issues that it could exacerbate. One should never overeat at any meal. Fruits can be taken at lunch or three hours after lunch.

In the evening, between 7 p.m. and 9 p.m., one can have light dinner when kapha is active. A good alternative is a few whole-wheat rotis (with ghee) and a vegetable, with possibly a cup of milk at the end. Or slices of fresh toasted bread with butter and hot soup or a bowl of pasta (without a lot of cream and cheese) and salad. Dinner should be simple, comprising one or two items that are light to digest as heavy meals are not recommended during kapha hours. We should not eat during pitta or vāta hours at night, as these are meant for sleep. We can, however, drink cooling liquids during pitta hours and clear the bladder before going to bed. A triphalā tea is a good option as it will balance all the doṣas and help with a good night's rest. It will also help to clear the bowels the next morning.

Ṛtucaryā

Variety is the spice of life. If it was summer all through the year, life would be tedious. Or if it snowed all the time, one would not appreciate it as much. Of course, it would be difficult, not just because of the impact on our mind, but also on the body. The different seasons allow us to tune into the rhythm of the time cycle and benefit from different ingredients and conditions throughout the year. Every season builds us in some way and we should take advantage of that.

While Dinacaryā delineates rules for daily conduct, Ṛtucaryā sets the rules for each season. According to Vāgabhaṭa, it refers to changes in diet and recreational activities as a result of seasons. Plants acquire the characteristics of the seasons in which they grow and then transmit that energy to those who consume them. Nature is programmed to produce foods that are beneficial when consumed in that season.

Earlier, we briefly discussed how vegetables with vāta prominence grow in the winter season. Winter causes dryness and cold, both the natures associated with vāta. The vegetables acquire these seasonal qualities as they grow. Now we tend to be lazy in such climates and the vāta from the vegetables supplies energy to fight that tendency. Besides, these vegetables carry a sweet taste (madhura rasa), tempting one to eat more. High digestive fire during those seasons helps digest the larger quantity of food easily.

The rule that we have visited repeatedly in the book is—eat whatever grows in that particular season. By following this rule, one also derives the maximum benefit from the seasons. Let's discuss the details of the rule we need to follow every season.

Movement of the Sun

There are three seasons when the sun travels in the northern direction and three in which it travels in the southern direction. Generally, as the sun travels north, the digestive fire (of those who live in India) goes down, and it gradually rises as the sun moves southward (Chart 4.1). This will not apply to a country like Australia, where the season pattern is opposite.

The first three seasons, when the sun moves in the northern direction (*uttarāyaṇa*), are late winter (*Śiriśa*), spring (*Vasanta*) and summer (*Griṣhma*). During these times, the heat of the sun gradually rises and dries everything as hot winds impede the cooling quality of the Earth. The result is that bitter, astringent and pungent tastes become prominent in the food that grows in these seasons. For example, neem trees blossom with fresh leaves, flowers and fruits. Similarly, the chilli pepper grows lavishly. The digestive fire in humans too slows down as the outside temperature increases (so that the body stays cool). Thus, nature supplies food that we would not feel attracted to. Food that grows naturally will slightly gain bitter, astringent or pungent tastes and people develop dryness within by eating such food. This is suitable to their low digestion fire. On the contrary, imagine what would happen if these seasons produced food that we would love to eat in more quantities (like those with sweet, salty and sour tastes)? We will tend to overeat and there will be a mismatch and a poor digestive fire cannot digest such food. In other words, if we eat food in summer that grew in winter, say cauliflower, from cold storages or by importing from cold regions, our stomach will find it difficult to digest. As a result we will suffer. So although the food with bitter, astringent and pungent taste is not contributing to our strength, it is just right for poor digestive fire and keeps us healthy. But if we don't follow the regimes ordained by mother nature, we will likely fall sick or feel uncomfortable. Of course, certain vegetables that grow on creepers, like spiny gourd (kantola), pointed gourd (paraval), bottle gourd (louki), etc., having sweet taste also appear. But these are very light and easy to digest (matching our low digestive fire). These vegetables are slightly bitter too. Sometimes bottle gourd may be too bitter to eat. I had experienced this sometimes when cooking for a large number of people.

So, nature supplies appropriate food to fight the harshness of these three seasons causing low digestive fire due to which the strength of the body gradually diminishes (Chart 4.1).

Chart 4.1: Ṛtucaryā—Digestive Fire during Various Seasons

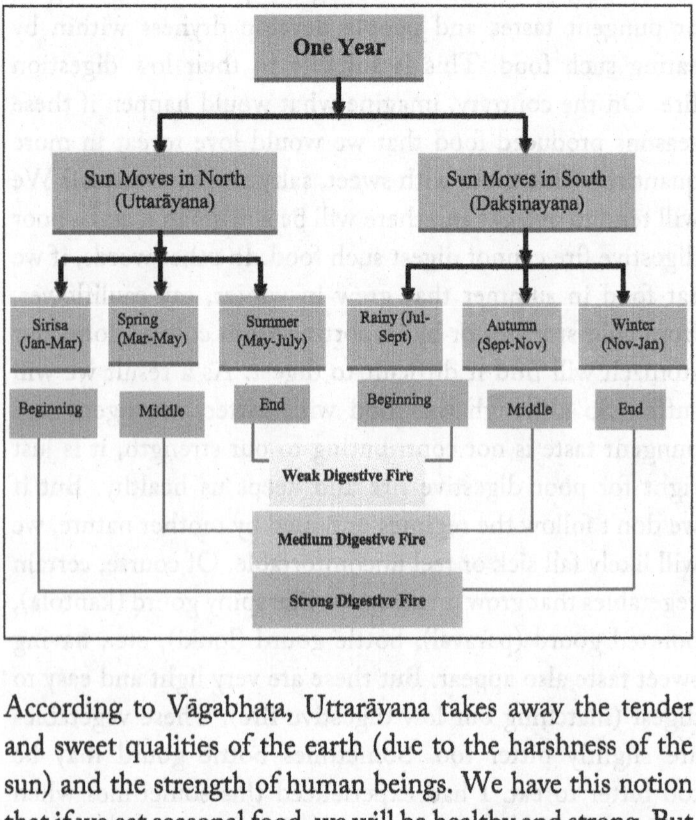

According to Vāgabhaṭa, Uttarāyana takes away the tender and sweet qualities of the earth (due to the harshness of the sun) and the strength of human beings. We have this notion that if we eat seasonal food, we will be healthy and strong. But during these seasons, by eating less we will be healthy for sure but not strong as we are in winter. But if we eat a lot of heavy food, ignoring the regime of these seasons, then we will be unhealthy, sick and weak too.

Those from Guntur district of Andhra Pradesh know that the best hot and pungent chillis are harvested and ripened during the hot summer. People from the heat belt of Andhra, Odisha, Maharashtra and Rajasthan partake of increased pungent tastes in their food. Highly pungent food will force one to eat less. Mexico, which is also on the hot belt of central America, is known for hot food containing chillis and jalapeño. You can observe this in some of the Thai and other south Asian cuisines (close to the equator). But if you are having the same cuisines in a different climate, please reduce the excess chillis. Yet, if you are from Mexico or Andhra and accustomed to hot preps and have developed the sātmya, then you may keep the chillis.

When the sun travels in the southern direction (*dakṣiṇayaṇa*), we experience the last three seasons, starting from monsoons (*Varṣā*), autumn (*Śarad*) and ending in winter (*Hemanta*). Due to the presence of rain clouds, cool winds and the coolness of the predominating moon, the digestive fire and bodily strength gradually grow to the maximum (Chart 4.1). Food with sour, salty and sweet tastes grows naturally during the rainy, autumn and winter seasons, respectively. For example, sweet taste is heavy and requires more digestive strength, which is available in winter. All kinds of sweet vegetables also grow during winter, blessed by moonshine. Thus in winter the bodily strength and sensory power increases to the maximum. One should minimize bitter and astringent food during these seasons as these tastes increase the vāta and dryness which is already high in the winter season.

Seasons and Doṣas: Different doṣas react differently in different seasons. One should learn to guard oneself from the imbalances by adjusting diet and lifestyle accordingly. Otherwise, the disturbed doṣas can lead to diseases. For example, kapha doṣa gradually increases during winter. Towards the end of the season, it will accumulate in the body. And during spring or early summer, it will start melting because of the heat of the rising sun. The trouble begins when it starts melting, leading to infections in the throat and sinus. At this time, we should regulate kapha-creating food, such as ice-cream, fruit custard with bananas, yoghurt and fruits with yoghurt. One must also cover oneself with warm clothing, especially the feet, head, ears and neck. This especially applies to people for whom kapha causes the main problem in their prakṛti. Similarly a pitta prakṛti person should strictly avoid indulging in pitta-creating food, such as excessively pungent food, hot spices and oily food during the monsoons (July–September in India) when the pitta starts to accumulate as a result of low digestive fire. One should avoid vāta-intensive food, such as chickpeas and black gram lentils during summer, when vāta accumulate easily due to low digestive fire. Again, this is truer for a vāta prakṛti person. This is explained in Table 4.3. We need to understand these principles and integrate them into our Dinacaryā or daily activities.

Table 4.3: Doṣa Imbalances in Different Seasons

Doṣa	Accumulates	Aggravates	Pacifies
Kapha	**Late Winter** (mid-Jan. to mid-Mar.) Avoid: Ice creams, sweets and kapha-increasing food	**Spring** (mid-Mar. to mid-May) Avoid: Ice creams, sweets and kapha-increasing food	**Summer** (mid-May to mid-Jul.) Regulated: kapha-increasing food
Pitta	**Rainy** (mid-Jul. to mid-Sep.) Avoid: Spicy, oily food	**Autumn** (mid-Sep. to mid-Nov.) Avoid: Spicy, oily food	**Winter** (mid-Nov. to mid-Jan.) Can be eaten: Spicy, oily food

Doṣa	Accumulates	Aggravates	Pacifies
Vāta	**Summer** (mid-May to mid-Jul.) Avoid: chickpeas, black gram, cheese and paneer, etc	**Rainy** (mid-Jul. to mid-Sep.) Avoid: chickpeas, black gram, cheese and paneer, etc	**Autumn** (mid-Sep. to mid-Nov.) Regulated: chickpeas, black gram, cheese and paneer, etc

Winter (Mid-November–Mid-March in India): In winter or Hemanta season, people are strong and the digestive fire is powerful. The digestive fire gets trapped in the body due to the chill outside, and as a result, there is greater hunger. Vāgabhaṭa says that the growing digestive fire starts consuming the tissues of the body with the help of wind or vāta in the body. So, one needs to eat all types of heavy food (cheese, paneer, beans and root vegetables) that is sour, salty and sweet to replenish the lost tissue. The strong digestive fire also allows one to eat to full satisfaction. Since the nights are longer in winter, one may feel hungry early in the morning, so it is a good idea to eat a heavier breakfast. People native to north India, especially in the winter, tend to eat heavy, rich and well-spiced food in breakfast this season. Vāgabhaṭa advises following this regime till of the end of Sirisha or mid-March.

During the few years I studied in the University of Delhi, I observed my hunger would rise like never before in winter. When I returned to Vrindavan (a three-hour drive from Delhi) nearly ten years later in winter, I could feel the same kind of hunger returning. Although it was not customary to eat a lot of rotis in Odisha, where I'm from, I remember happily munching on rotis with palak paneer in winters, and digesting the same effortlessly.

Spring (Mid-March–Mid-May in India): Because of the rising sun, the accumulated kapha from winter starts melting in spring. This can lead to many diseases. Therefore, the kapha needs to be controlled swiftly. Also, as the heat rises, the digestive fire slows down to keep the body cool from the inside. Spring onwards, one should eat food that is dry (anti kapha), with cooling potency (ash gourd for example) and is easy to digest. Aged barley, wheat, and mango juice mixed with cardamom, mint and honey are also recommended. One should also put oil in the nasal cavity periodically under the guidance of an Ayurvedic doctor. As the temperature rises, one should considerably reduce kapha-creating heavy and hot potent food that is fatty, sour and sweet (in general hard to digest). It is best to be in a cool area during the day.

Summer (Mid-May–Mid-July in India): In summer, the rays of the sun become stronger, and it appears to destroy everything. Our digestive strength is not spared either. The strength of kapha diminishes and vāta keeps increasing. So, food that is hot in potency, pungent and sour, as well as heavy physical exercise and exposure to the sun should be avoided. One should partake of food that is sweet, fatty but light to digest, and cool in potency. Food in liquid form, such as soup, is beneficial. White rice with moong beans and vegetables growing in creepers, such as ridged gourd, is good for the body. Pastries/pies/bread made from corn flour are also all right to consume during the evenings. Corn grows during these months in India.

Monsoons (Mid-July–Mid-September in India): In India, summer is followed by rain. The already debilitated digestive fire is further affected because of dark clouds and the sudden advent of cold air with hail or water. Rain cools down the weather but the moisture also traps the heat, creating hot, humid conditions.

As a result, the digestive fire is also low during this time. And because of too many changes, all the doṣas go out of balance. Thus, it is recommended that one maintain a diet of very light food, consisting of grains, pulses, fats and vegetables. Grains should be aged well (about a year).

Autumn (Mid-September–Mid-November in India): The pitta doṣa that accumulates in our bodies during the rainy season greatly aggravates in autumn due to sudden exposure to sunlight, after the clouds clear. It is best to eat easily digested food such as moong and pointed gourd. Moong also has an astringent taste, which balances pitta.

Table 4.4 summarizes the recommended dietary regime during different seasons. One should transition from one type of diet to another from the last week of the preceding season to the end of the first week of the succeeding season.

Table 4.4: Dietary Regime for Various Seasons

Season	Affected Doṣa	Tastes Recommended	Recommended Regime
Rainy	Pitta	Sweet, Salty and Sour	Light easy to digest, include cooling diets towards the end of the season
Autumn	Pitta	Sweet, Bitter, Astringent	Light dry food. Sweet balances pitta, bitter astringent helps keep the diet light

Season	Affected Doṣa	Tastes Recommended	Recommended Regime
Winter	None	Sweet, Salty and Sour	Heavy and good quantity
Śiriśa (end of winter)	Kapha	Sweet, Salty and Sour	Guard against Kapha
Spring	Kapha	Bitter, Pungent, Astringent	Dry food. Naturally present in astringent food like plantains and pomegranate
Summer	Pitta	Sweet	Light meals, cooling drink

How Do We Recognize the Onset of a Season?

We need to be vigilant about our surroundings to sense changes in seasons early on. Seasons appear differently in different parts of the world. It rains throughout the year in countries such as the UK. But because of the cold weather, this rain doesn't affect people the same way the monsoon affects those living in India. During monsoons in India, the heat and the sun will affect the pitta doṣa, but rain in the UK and the US won't have the same effect.

In places like Malaysia, it rains every day in the late afternoon, while the sun is high in the sky. This is usually unchanged every day as it is close to the equator. It affected my pitta badly because it was as though I was experiencing summer and monsoons at the same time.

Thanks to my international travels to teach sāttvic cooking, I have learnt traditions and habits to perfectly deal with different seasons. But these beautiful traditions of local customs have not been preserved everywhere over generations. As a result, we are confused about how to fix ourselves and interact with the environment. But it's time to return to that tradition-based knowledge and rectify our diet and lifestyles. If we can observe the impact of seasons on our tridoṣa and make the corresponding adjustments in our diet, we will achieve a lot. I am sure it will not be difficult to ascertain the regime one needs to follow.

In some parts of India, because of its geographical location, one can experience all the six seasons. But towards the north, in the Himalayas, the winter is longer, so one may miss Śiriśa or late winter. Similarly, in western countries, the winter is longer. Every part of the world has its own traditions, and a lot can be learnt from local traditions and used to fine-tune one's Ayurvedic knowledge and application of it.

Conclusion

In this section we discussed the science that regulates our digestion and the factors that control digestion from within and without. We also discussed the eight golden rules that we need to follow, and contradict unhealthy combinations of items.

In the following section titled 'Yogi Plate' we will focus on two aspects of these eight rules—Karana or the cooking process and the Upabhoktā or the consumer. We will return to our focus on sāttvic cooking and lifestyle.

Section Five

Yogi Plate

Food, Mind and Digestion
Be Your Own Favourite Cook!
Qualifications of a Cook
Cooking
Recipes and Cooking Methods
The Right Method of Serving and Eating
Conduct after Eating

Yogi Plate

'You don't have to cook fancy or complicated masterpieces—just good food from fresh ingredients.'

—Julia Child

Earlier, people would *walk* to their workplace, the market, their relatives' houses, friends, etc. We were a lot less dependent on machines. Even household chores required more muscle power, such as washing clothes, drawing water from a well or a river and bringing it home, milling flour, pounding spices, removing the husk from rice grains, grinding soaked grains for batter, chopping vegetables for a family of 10–20 people, cooking, cleaning the dishes, etc. So, generally, all these activities would result in a productive exercise. But thanks to mechanization, such activities require a lot less muscle power. However, our bodies have remained the same and need exercise to stay healthy. In this modern scenario, we have to find extra time for exercise as our work no longer includes it. Modern lifestyles have also given rise to many complicated anxieties. We need exercises that resolve our body's quota of exercise as well as those that relax our mind.

During my yoga teacher training programme, the most difficult part was to relax the mind as and when instructed by the teacher. The āsanas thought difficult can be improved with practice but relaxing the mind requires more mastery. I have realized that it becomes tougher as we age. Yoga, which also involves exercise of the mind, should be included in our daily regime. Just as food is classified as being in three modes—sāttvic, rājasic and tāmasic—exercise is also categorized into three modes. Yoga is a sāttvic exercise that nourishes both the body and the mind. Walking early in the morning is a sāttvic practice too, especially if the surroundings are scenic. Weight lifting, athletics, jogging, and martial art are rājasic exercises, in the mode of passion. This is essential for people engaged in security and military services.

Sports and adventure activities involving risks to our life such as bungee jumping and car racing are considered tāmasic exercises. Just as sāttvic food is universally recommended, yoga is recommended for all. Even a person who does strenuous exercise should practise yoga to have control over the body and mind. Power, prestige and popularity, associated with passion, can influence one's mind negatively with pride and envy. But a sāttvic lifestyle centred on the practice of yoga, meditation and sāttvic food helps us focus on the right purpose. This however, does not mean one should give up exercise that one enjoys, such as boxing, running or martial arts.

Exercise without a proper diet is futile and vice versa. Yoga and sāttvic diet are intimately related. While more people across the world have begun to practise yoga, diets the world over seem to have deteriorated. This has minimized the benefits of yoga as well.

In general, people are reluctant to change or regulate their diet. The mouth is the gateway to preserving one's life. So we should never compromise on what we put into it. But food is also a primary source of pleasure. So this clash creates a fear about regulations. Will I have to sacrifice my French fries? Do I really have to give up my cherished food? We should know that Ayurvedic sāttvic cooking does not end at Indian cuisine. If we understand the principles, we can apply it to any cuisine and not miss anything. Sāttvic and Ayurvedic principles will guide the recipes, the timing and quantity.

The main purpose of this book is to understand and apply the pure sāttvic concepts to our existing diet and make it suitable for our lifestyle. Any person who understands the importance of sāttvic diet and wants to practise it will benefit from the advice in this section. One of the best benefits of sāttvic food is it has a calming effect on the digestive system as well as on the mind. The digestive system can affect the mind and the mind can affect the digestive system. Let's discuss the influence of the mind over digestion which is a primary concern for a yogi aspiring for a long healthy life.

Food, Mind and Digestion

Besides following daily and seasonal regimes, you should also be aware of your own internal seasons. In particular, your mind goes through various hot and cold phases over the course of a day and life. And when the mind's temperature changes, your digestive fire also gets affected.

One of my yoga instructors, Robert Sankara Moses, taught me a lesson that is imprinted in my heart. He spoke of a deer who was fearlessly grazing on green grass till a lion appeared. Among all of the deer's friends, the lion decided to focus on him. At that very moment, the deer stopped eating. Its digestive system stopped working, and its heart began to beat fast.

Everyone has two nervous systems. One is voluntary, which controls activities such as the writing of this book, and the other is involuntary, which controls activities such as the beating of the heart, working of the lungs and also digestion. The involuntary or autonomous nervous system does not care for our instructions. It acts only to protect the body and has no other boss. So, when the deer sensed an imminent attack, the digestive system stopped. All the blood supply and energy was focused on escaping. It was not time to eat; it was time to run the hell out of there. The deer's heart, another involuntary nervous system, started pumping heavily even before the deer decided to run, supplying all the necessary energy to help it pick up speed. So, the deer ran for its life as the lion zeroed in on him. The powerful lion pounced and gripped the poor deer's neck in its jaws, but the deer was still breathing. At that very moment, the lion heard the loud sound of a gunshot, and ran for its own life, dropping the deer. The deer miraculously escaped death. But somehow, the traumatic experience was so intense that the digestive system wouldn't restart! The poor deer was in total fear and walked around trying to munch the same fresh lush green grass and drink clean water from the lake, but the stomach would have none of it. The deer eventually died after struggling for twenty-five days.

This story teaches us how our digestive system is connected to our stress levels. Anger, frustration, intense greed, depression, jealousy and envy take us away from our digestive system. The impact is proportionate to the extent of the negative emotion we are afflicted with. All of us have some experience of this. For example, while mourning the passing away of a dear one, people are advised to eat simple food for ten days, because in mourning, the mind and stomach cannot handle rich luxurious food.

In the above example, with the surging energy provided by the sympathetic nervous system, the deer had two choices: either to fight the lion or run away. Just imagine if the deer wouldn't do either and just stood there stupefied, the excess high blood pressure, if not released, would destroy the brain or the heart. This is exactly what happens to modern human beings in stressful situations. For example, when one is having a tough time with a boss, spouse or a dear friend, one cannot escape and run or fight with them. The result is increased blood pressure and harm to our health. Of course, no one thinks of eating at such moments and may take to alcohol/drugs or self-destructive behaviour. In such situations, try to go for a long walk or exercise instead, while focusing on the positive aspects of life, and internally calming down.

The mind has to calm down. Anger and frustration will not help. So, focusing on a higher purpose and taking every event as an opportunity to grow, one should give up anger and frustration. Sadness is a sign of ignorance. Feeling hungry and relishing a meal is a sign of good health. In a family life, make the home such a happy place through love and sacrifice that all the outside stress dissolves the moment you enter the home.

Dejection and failure have a deep impact on the mind, and in turn affect digestion. So the best ways to counter challenges in life is to practise positivity, develop resilience to absorb personal defeat and learn to move on to newer projects and opportunities. In other words, there has to be a certain level of detachment from the results of our activities. Detachment comes when there is a higher goal in mind. For example, when a team is participating in a championship, they may lose a league match but they still have some chances of reaching the finals. Failure in one match will not hold us back if we are focused on the championship. But focusing on the loss will make winning even the next league match difficult. Pride or overconfidence can affect us negatively too when we win a league match, preventing us from focusing on the goal. So, detachment is necessary to keep stress at bay.

The struggle to conquer the mind is not new, and most great thinkers and sages recommend meditation. Training the mind thus will also have a great impact on the digestive system and iron out kinks in its functioning. So, try to make time for meditation every day.

If stress affects digestion, it is clear that there is a strong connection between the mind and the digestive system. This means that the digestive system can also affect the mind. Sāttvic food helps one's mind develop sāttvic qualities. Ayurveda says that rajas and tamas or passion and ignorance are doṣas (faults) of the mind and are the root causes of all sickness. On the other hand, sattva brings purity to the mind. Sāttvic food and lifestyle has an important role to play in bringing an element of truth to all levels of social intercourse.

Be Your Own Favourite Cook!

When I started to live in the ashram of the Radha Gopinath Temple of Mumbai, many well-wishing friends started inviting me to their homes for dinner. My mind and heart would fill with happiness, but my body would often fail to appreciate the gesture. A city like Mumbai, with a population of 20 million, has families from different cultures. The food, although fresh and healthy, would not suit my nature and was asātmya (not sātmya). It only reaffirmed the importance of cooking my own food most of the time. Because the cook who knows my nature best is me! No one knows me better than I do myself. Usually, apart from us, the person who knows us best is our mother, as we are an extension of her body, her compassion and her sacrifice.

Your nature dictates the quantity of salt and spices you will like, which grain is right, which oil and which vegetables suit you, etc. Your nature directs you to cook what will suit you the best. All you need is some skill, which gets refined as you keep cooking. A person who can eat can learn to cook too. Do visit my website (www.yogiplate.com) to learn more on Ayurvedic sāttvic cooking skills. We will be happy to assist. The more we practise cooking with happiness, the better we will be at it.

Skills apart, the challenge to cook a perfect sāttvic meal is your own state of mind. Because sāttvic food has to nourish the mind, a good deal of subtlety is involved in cooking sāttvic food. This requires much more than just sāttvic ingredients, it requires a sāttvic mind.

One day in college, I missed dinner while studying late in the library. The hostel mess had shut by the time I left the library. I was not sure where to eat. As I was heading back, a friend joined me and invited me to have dinner with him at the mess! He said he had asked one cook to wait for him. As he was the mess secretary, the cook had obliged. I agreed, but upon reaching the mess I noticed that the cook wasn't too happy to see me. He was expecting one customer and two appeared. I could understand, after a whole day's load of work, it's difficult to handle surprises. I ate the dinner and thanked both of them.

Later I thought, if my mother were there, she would have happily cooked for both of us. When your loved one cooks for you, they tend to do so with natural affection that nourishes the heart, mind and body. This is not always the case when a stranger is cooking for us.

Thus, the tradition exists of sādhus and yogis preferring to cook their own food. As far as our own mind is concerned, the better we do our spiritual sādhanā, the better we will be at it.

When I lived at the ashram, I was trained to chant mantras that are meant to purify the mind. But there are proper procedures and training required to chant these mantras so that they are more effective. Just as there are procedures for a proper bath to purify the body (rinsing, scrubbing with mud and herbs and finally washing off thoroughly), similarly, there are certain rules to chant the mantras. This includes sitting straight, controlling your breathing and steadily focusing on the vibrations of the mantras.

Qualifications of a Cook

Normally a list of qualifications is required to enter any stream of training. But since food is an inseparable part of us, the only prerequisite is a desire to cook. The rest can all be refined.

To maintain good cooking quality, one needs to follow standard practices. For example, cleanliness is one of the most important aspects of cooking. Keeping a tidy mind is even more important. One should, for example, enter a kitchen after bathing, as it not only cleanses the body but also refreshes our mind. Similarly, meditation and chanting of mantras delivers the mind from many impurities that might have been deposited from many lifetimes, lurking somewhere, deep in the subconscious. These may pop up on our mind's valley from time to time and contaminate our cooking.

In case of people who usually cook for the entire family, the impurities take a back seat because of the overpowering selfless love and affection they usually put into the cooking.

Yogis, according to the Bhagavad Gitā, focus their mind on God (*Parmātmā*) in their own heart while chanting the mantras. So bathing, wearing fresh clothes, meditation, worships of gods, our forefathers and spiritual masters cleanses the body and the consciousness.

In my humble journey as a cook, I have had many chances to cook for my friends, family, guests, as well as deities at temples, spiritual masters and thousands of strangers. Most often, people would appreciate the food, but they would rarely appreciate the cook. However, when I cooked for my spiritual master, His Holiness Radhanath Swami, he called me and appreciated me as he was appreciating the food. That was a unique unforgettable experience, and it was so fulfilling that I felt proud to be a cook.

Cooking

Cooking can be a great recreational activity. To keep yourself absorbed, listen to some sāttvic music, an inspirational talk or an educational lesson while you cook. This way your mind will be satisfied as you get a feeling of gaining something.

Planning: Ideally, the menu should be planned in advance as it saves a lot of time. Plan a menu based on the season, available vegetables and how you are feeling. If cooking for a family, one needs to look after all others' needs as well. Suppose you want to cook minestrone soup or rajma (kidney beans), make sure you soak the beans for eight hours. Similarly, if you plan to make samosas in the evening, boil a few potatoes for the stuffing while cooking lunch. Planning keeps the mind peaceful and balanced during cooking. It is important that we are not anxious during the process. If all the ingredients and spices are not in place, it will lead to irritation, and it will be tougher to maintain a sattva and positive frame of mind.

Executing: The steps of the recipe should be clear in our mind, like a singer who knows the lyrics to a well-practised song. But memorizing the lyrics and actually singing them is completely different. It's important to feel the words while performing the song and make sure they are in harmony with the music. So, while the recipe should be clear in the mind, it needs to merge with the ingredients in front of you.

It's important to maintain tidiness while cooking. Think of baking a cake. The kitchen should not look as if a bomb went off in it and a beautiful cake appeared from nowhere! Sounds familiar?

Keeping the kitchen clean is a way of respecting it. The kitchen, in Vedic tradition, is considered no less than the altar of God. Because the food that comes out of the kitchen is called 'naivedya', an offering for the pleasure of the Lord. So, the sanctity of the kitchen is utmost. One of my friends, who was serving with me in the ashram and who did his Masters in Hotel Management, taught me the golden rule to keep the kitchen clean. In hotel industries, they call it CYG, clean as you go. Yes, cooking and cleaning should go on simultaneously. Then our mind and that of anyone else in the kitchen will be at peace too. And it ensures that you aren't left with an arduous task at the end of the cooking. Practise this every time you cook and you will thank my friend for the advice.

*

Ideally, an Ayurvedic meal should include all the six rasas or tastes in one meal. The combination will depend upon the season. In this section, I will include six recipes, each corresponding prominently to one rasa or taste.

In one of my favourite places of worship, Mayapur, birthplace of Lord Caitanya, I learnt how to cook a perfect

Bengali meal from a monk named Sasanka Prabhu. He has been cooking this meal expertly for the past three decades and makes sure it comprises all six rasas. In his honour, I would like to present six recipes here. I have included plant-based alternatives for vegans.

Finding the Right Cooking Pots

Clay pots are considered the best for cooking. In Jagannath Puri, most of the food is still cooked in clay pots. You must pay a visit and taste the khichri and dali prasād at the temple there.

The clay pots they use are raw and uncoated, and used only once. Clay pots are not reused unless the pot is used for roasting, as food particles enter the tiny pores in the clay and cannot be cleaned. These pots cost very little, are environment friendly and help cook very tasty food. Nowadays, some shops sell coated clay pots, so that they can be reused. These are not as good for cooking. Cooking clay pots are to be used only once, unless they are being used for roasting.

For sturdier utensils, it's best to look for them in kansa copper and cast iron. But the world over, people have abandoned these cooking pots and switched to cheap coated and lightweight aluminium pots or stainless steel pots. The aluminum wears off while cooking and can contaminate the food when we cook in such pots. Aluminium is not known to have any physiological impact; however, because of its atomic size and electric charge, it is sometimes a competitive inhibitor of several essential elements with similar characteristics, such as magnesium, calcium and iron. While stainless steel is harmless, it doesn't add to the cooking quality nor is it a good conductor of heat. That means a typical stainless steel pot heats only on the bottom and may burn or over cook the food at the bottom of the pot. Aluminium is a very good conductor of heat, but makes the food āma. Also avoid aluminium cans, foil/wraps, etc.

Iron is heavy and prone to rust, but if used daily, it will not be an issue. Do make sure to wipe and wash the pan before using, so that any rust that may have formed is removed. Or oil the pan after washing and wipe off the oil before using the utensil again. Iron is an extremely good conductor of heat, which cooks the food well. It adds to the taste too.

Whichever pots you use, make sure the material is thick and sturdy. The low-cost thin metallic pots are not good for cooking properly as they will burn the food at the point of contact. The pot has to cook the ingredients by supplying heat and at the same time protect them from the fire.

Pressure cookers raise the temperature beyond 100°C, which is not natural for food ingredients and thus may reduce the prāṇa-śakti by a good deal. In my experience, cooking in an open pot is much healthier and results in much tastier food than pressurized cooking. Many who have switched over to open-pot cooking have reported the same to me. Even chickpeas and kidney beans can be cooked in open pots, but they just need to cook for longer over a steady flame and with enough water. We have cooked chole very often in open pots to feed over 5000 pilgrims in holy places like Vrindavan.

In Punjab, black gram is traditionally cooked on a low wood fire all night long. The heat would provide warmth to the home during the winter night and cook the dal so well that it gave strength, health and happiness. Of course, one needs to be careful with fire when it is on all night. Usually, it's not a live fire but charcoal that lasts all night. My father used to bake cheesecake (from fresh paneer) on a low fire all night. The taste was unmatched and unforgettable.

Cooking Fire

Wood-fired pizzas have become popular all over the world now. This is because wood fire burns steadily, and the temperature of the fire is not very intense, rather diffused. It also creates a good amount of moisture and smoke. In a wood-fired pizza oven, the pizza cooks well on the stone and becomes crisp on the bottom, but remains moist on the top due to the moisture generated by the wood fire. During digestion, which is akin to cooking, kapha doṣa provides the moisture. Without the moisture, the pizza will be dry on top. Besides, the smoke from the wood enhances the flavour. A steady low fire preserves the prāṇa-śakti or vitality of the food.

Liquefied petroleum gases or clean gases are very intense in heat and create little moisture, but are the next best choice. Electric heated plates provide intense heating and no moisture at all. A microwave just causes the water molecules in the food to vibrate and dries the food directly. Considering modern amenities and lifestyles, you may not have access to a wood fire. In that case, try to opt for cooking over an LPG flame over electric hot plates or microwave ovens. Most of the following recipes have been tried over LPG fire and cooked in traditional pots.

Recipes and Cooking Methods

Here I have provided sample recipes with some Ayurvedic understanding. I will also try to explain the intricate principles associated with sāttvic cooking.

Raw Food/Salads

Salads, usually served raw, are ready to eat food, and thus a lot of precautions should be taken in terms of hygiene and cleanliness during preparation. The cooked items pass through a fire-purification process and thus are safer for human consumption. But we need to be extra careful while eating raw salad, especially in a hot and humid climate (like that of India) as the bacteria load can easily catch up. A salad has to be served fresh. And as mentioned earlier, the dressing aids in digestion. Usually, it has a prominent sour and pungent taste. In the first dressing, it is orange juice and pepper and in the second dressing, it is lemon juice and black pepper. Olive oil helps to balance the vāta doṣa.

Lettuce with Orange Dressing

Ingredients:

Salad

1 grated carrot
1 chopped iceberg lettuce
¼ cup sliced olives
2 cups rocket leaves
2 tbsp chopped celery stalks
½ tsp fresh lemon juice
3 tsp extra virgin olive oil
2 tbsp chopped basil leaves

Dressing 1: Orange Dressing

⅓ cup boiled cashew nuts
2 cups orange juice
2 tbsp brown sugar
4 tbsp extra virgin olive oil
½ tsp salt
½ tsp black pepper powder
1 tbsp nutritional yeast

Dressing 2:

2 tsp fresh lemon juice
2 tsp extra-virgin olive oil
¼ tsp black pepper powder
1 green chilli chopped fine (optional)
1 tsp salt

Directions:

- Wash all the salad ingredients with cool clean water. Washing increases the freshness and prāṇa of the salad.

Dry the leaves using a drier. Peel and grate the carrot into fine shreds. Chop the celery into fine slices.

- Mix all the above ingredients with the remaining ingredients listed in the salad category. Stir it by gently tossing the ingredients up and down.

Dressing:

Choose from any of the two dressings. In a blender, put all the ingredients listed under the selected dressing. Make sure the cashew nuts are at room temperature. Fresh fragrant orange juice is preferable over packaged juices. Blend the ingredients to a smooth consistency.

Serve the lettuce salad with a small bowl of orange or lemon dressing.

Cooked Food

The following list comprises cooked dishes based on different rasas/tastes.

Sweet, Salty & Pungent

1. Khichri: Rice and Lentils with Vegetables
2. Eggplant Pakoras
3. Palak Paneer Paratha: Spinach Stuffed Paratha

Sour, Salty and Pungent

1. Pineapple Chutney
2. Buttermilk

Bitter and Astringent

1. Sukto: Bittermelon, plantains, raw papaya in mustard sauce

1. Khichri: Rice and Lentils with Vegetables (Sweet)

Khichri, also known as Khichdi, is a balanced wholesome preparation that is cooked throughout India. The fact that it is cooked all over shows its universal nature. It is healthy as well as tasty! Rice, lentils and vegetables are cooked together. It has all the nutrients a meal can offer—carbohydrates, proteins and minerals. It also balances all the three doṣas and can be eaten at any time of the day and any season. The spices need to be adjusted for people of different prakṛti or in case of imbalanced doṣa.

Ingredients[*]

½ cup rice
½ cup moong dal
7 cups water
½ cup bottle gourd (small cubes) or zucchini
¼ cup carrots (small cubes)
½ cup green beans (chopped ½ inch long)
¾ cup red pumpkin (diced ½ inch)
¼ cup fresh peas (to be avoided if vāta is high)
1-½ cup spinach (washed and chopped)

---

[*] Vegetables that grow on creepers, sweet in taste and are light to digest are preferred. Some root vegetables such as carrots can make the khichri heavy, but it is fine to eat them in winter. In summer and rainy season, one should avoid root vegetables.

Tadka (Spicing)

2 tbsp extra virgin olive oil/ahimsā ghee

1 tsp pancha phodan (equal proportion of mustard seeds, fennel seeds and cumin seeds and half portion of fenugreek seeds and kalonji seeds)

¼ tsp asafoetida powder

¼ tsp turmeric powder

4–5 curry leaves (fresh or dried)

½ tsp ginger (chopped fine)

1 tsp salt

2 tbsp chopped cilantro leaves

Directions:

- Wash the rice and dal separately and soak them in water. Boil the water in a heavy-bottomed pot. Make sure the pot can hold three times the water already in it.
- Add the soaked dal.
- Start cutting vegetables in the order and shapes mentioned in the list of ingredients. Wash and drain the water.
- Keep adding the vegetables as you cut them, except spinach. Then add the soaked rice (about fifteen minutes after adding the lentils). Cook it all together for twenty to twenty-five minutes over a high flame while stirring time to time to make sure it doesn't stick to the bottom. Make sure the rice grains don't break while stirring. Cook till the dish has a thick consistency.
- Lower the flame. Add chopped spinach. Stir in the salt. Cover with a lid.

Spicing:

Heat oil in a thick-bottomed pot. Add the spices in the order as given in the list of ingredients.* Make sure the whole spices like mustard seeds crack open and asafoetida cooks well. When the ginger turns brownish, add the turmeric powder. Add the tadka to the boiling khichri. Stir nicely. Cook for a few minutes. Switch off the fire and stir in the chopped cilantro. Serve with molten ahimsa ghee, spiced yoghurt and roasted papad.

2. Eggplant Pakoras (Salty)

Eggplants, according to Kṣema Śarmā, author of *Kṣema-kutuhalam*, stimulate the taste buds, help ignite gastric fire,

* Cooking spices properly makes a preparation tasty and healthy too. Overly cooked spices will lose their benefits and undercooked spices will not yield the benefits. Whole spices, like mustard seeds, etc. require hot oil/ghee to split open and provide the essence our digestive environment needs. Among these spices, there are seeds that are tough to crack open (mustard, fenugreek seeds), some that are not as difficult (coriander seeds) and some that easily crack open (like cumin seeds). One needs to add the tough ones to the heated oil first. Make sure the oil heats enough to open these seeds. The moment it touches the oil, it should crack open like mini fire crackers. As the temperature drops, add the softer seeds, such as cumin seeds. It should be done in quick succession. When the cumin seeds crack open, lower the flame and sprinkle the asafoetida powder. Wet spices such as curry leaves and ginger paste are added next. Wet spices bring down the temperature of oil considerably and should never be added before the whole seeds and asafoetida. After the addition of the wet spices, the heat can be increased. When the ginger turns brown, powdered spices, such as turmeric, which are easiest to cook, are added. Care must be taken not to burn the powdered spices. The whole combination is then added to the main preparation, be it khichri or dal (lentil soup) or vegetable stew. These principles can be followed for all kinds of spicing.

mitigate vāta, support heart functions, increase semen production and are light or easily digested.

Organic eggplants of all colours are very tasty when cooked in ghee and spiced with sautéed asafoetida and black pepper.

This crispy savoury can be eaten during late afternoon when the vāta is high and also goes well with khichri during lunch. It kindles digestive fire and puts away anorexia.

Ingredients:
2 medium-sized eggplants
1 tsp salt
½ tsp turmeric

Batter
1 cup chickpea flour
¼ tsp carom seeds
¼ tsp asafoetida powder
⅛ tsp turmeric powder
½ tsp saindha salt
Water

Use cold pressed oil for deep-frying (sesame oil or ghee for all seasons, mustard for winter, and coconut oil for summer)

Chat Masala for Dressing on Top
Combine 1 tsp roasted cumin powder, ¼ tsp freshly crushed black pepper powder, ¼ tsp black salt and ¼ tsp dried mango powder.

Directions:

- Wash and slice the eggplants into 3 mm discs. Rub salt and turmeric on them and keep them aside.

Batter

Mix all the dry ingredients with a clean, dry hand. Add a little water and beat it till you have a thick paste without any trapped balls of dry flour. Beat it for a few minutes until it is smooth. Add a little more water to dilute it to a homemade yoghurt consistency or a little thinner than cake batter.

Frying

Heat oil in a deep flat thick iron pot. Just two inches deep of oil is enough for frying. Drain all the water from the marinated eggplant without squeezing. Keep the batter close to where the oil is heating. Then dip each piece of eggplant in the batter, bring it as close as possible to the surface of the oil and drop it in. Do not drop from a height to avoid the oil splashing. The oil should not be too hot (then it will fry the outer layer too quickly, and the inner portion will be raw) and the oil should not be cold either, as that would make the pakoras soggy and oily. The right temperature is when the coating crisps up as soon as it touches the oil. The eggplant pieces will be cooked when the tiny water bubbles around the pakoras nearly disappear, and the coating is golden yellow or light brown. Upon removing the discs, the oil should drain and dry off quickly. Sprinkle chat masala and serve hot.

Never cover the pakoras with a lid, especially when they are hot, for it will catch moisture quickly and become soggy. Keep it uncovered and serve before it cools down.

3. Palak Paneer Paratha: Spinach Stuffed Paratha (Sweet and Astringent)

This should be eaten during winter or by people with good strength of digestive fire, as it is heavy to digest. This can be served during lunch and as a winter breakfast or dinner. Spinach is sweet as well as slightly astringent. Paneer is sweet and unctuous and wheat is wholesome and easy to digest. Replace paneer with soft tofu if you are vegan and great millet flour (jawāri atta) if you are gluten-intolerant. Spices like asafoetida and black pepper will regulate the vāta creating potency of spinach. People with vāta imbalance should avoid this stuffed paratha or eat less of it.

Ingredients:

Dough
2 cups wholewheat flour
½ tsp saindhava (rock) salt
Hot boiling water (nearly ¾ cup)

Stuffing
2 cups fresh ahimsa milk or ½ cup crumbled soft tofu
500 gm (1 pound) spinach
½ tsp saindha salt
¼ tsp asafoetida powder
¼ tsp freshly crushed pepper powder
¼ cup sliced olives (optional)

Ghee or extra virgin olive oil for cooking

Directions:

- Make a medium soft dough by combing flour and salt and then adding the boiling hot water. Boiling water cooks the wheat and makes it lighter to digest. Use a spoon to mix the hot water, and when it starts to cool down a bit, use your palm to knead the dough.
- To prepare the paneer, bring the milk to boiling point and switch off the fire. Add clear lemon juice while gently stirring the milk in one direction. As soon as the cheese separates, cease adding the lemon juice. Excess heating and addition of juice renders the cheese hard. Using a thin cheese cloth, separate the cheese and wash it with cool water. Squeeze the excess water out.
- Blanche the spinach in boiling water for 5–10 minutes. Do not cover the spinach with a lid to avoid discolouring. Drain, cool and chop the spinach. Again, using your palms, squeeze out the excess water. If not squeezed, you will not be able to roll the paratha as the stuffing will be too wet.
- Mix the salt, spices, olives slices, chopped dry spinach and dried paneer/tofu together gently to make the stuffing.
- Divide the dough as well as the stuffing into six to eight balls. The stuffing should be the same size as the dough. Flatten the dough and place the stuffing on it. Then, using your palms, close and seal the stuffing from all sides. Roll this ball and cook it on a flat cast iron pan with ghee/olive oil. While roasting, using a flat spoon to press down the paratha so that the steam puffs the paratha and cooks it nicely from inside as the oil cooks it from outside. Cut it into four and serve with spiced churned yoghurt or green chutney.

4. Pineapple Chutney (Sour and Pungent)

This sour preparation should not be eaten in excess. This prep enhances the taste and increase the process of digestion. It is inspired by the traditional cooking at Jagannath Puri. Although pineapple is a pitta enhancer, the use of jaggery and coconut in this item makes it pitta pacifying.

Ingredients:

One ripe pineapple
½ cup grated fresh coconut
¼ cup dry raisins
¼ cup organic jaggery powder
1-¼ tsp saindhava (rock) salt
⅛ tsp turmeric
1 tsp ginger paste
1 tsp mango-flavoured ginger (āmbakasi adā in Odiya, ambāhalud in Maharashtra, etc.)
2-½ cups water

Seasoning:
1 tbsp ghee/extra virgin olive oil
¼ tsp mustard seeds
¼ tsp fenugreek seeds
¼ tsp asafoetida powder
4–6 fresh curry leaves
½ tsp lemon juice
1 tbsp chopped fresh cilantro

Directions:

- Wash, peel and remove the stalk and the eyes of the pineapple. Dice into small cubes (¼ inch). Then put all the ingredients (except jaggery and ingredients listed under seasoning) in a thick-bottomed pot, along with the chopped pineapple and bring it to a boil. Cook until the pineapple softens and partially dissolves into the gravy. Add the jaggery and cook for a few more minutes.
- Heat ghee in a small pot just below the smoke point. Add the mustard and fenugreek seeds so that they sputter. Lower the fire and sauté the asafoetida powder till it turns brownish. Then quickly add the fresh curry leaves before the asafoetida burns. Add this to the cooking pineapple and turn off the flame. Stir in the lemon juice and fresh cilantro.

Fenugreek is bitter and usually used in all sour items as an antidote to balance the pitta.

5. Buttermilk

Balances all the doṣas. To be avoided during the rainy season. Also when pitta is in excess.

Ingredients:

1 cup fresh yoghurt from cow milk (ahimsā)
½ cup chilled potable mineral water
1 tsp saindhava (rock) salt
A pinch of asafoetida
½ tsp freshly roasted cumin powder

½ tsp rock candy sugar powder
1 tsp finely chopped fresh mint leaves (pudinā)

Directions:

- Churn the yoghurt with a quarter cup chilled water using a hand churning rod (manthni or Ravi in Hindi). Churning is done usually in the morning when the temperature is cool. Churn for 15–20 minutes. Add the remaining chilled water. The butter will float on the surface. An electric hand blender also effectively removes butter. But they affect the prāṇa-śakti. Remove the butter and add all the remaining ingredients to the buttermilk. Churn for a few minutes more before serving.
- Vegans may supplement their diet with kombucha (a drink produced by fermenting sweet tea with yeast and bacteria).
- This is beneficial for gut culture, but its effect on tridoṣa, which may depend on the extent of fermentation, needs to be evaluated.

6. Sukto (Bitter and Astringent)

Dr Vasant Lad, a prolific author on Ayurveda, says bitter is better. Sukto, although bitter, tastes excellent. The plantain in the ingredient adds to the astringent taste. This preparation balances kapha, vāta and pitta. It should be served with plain steamed rice. The spices used are a mixture of mustard seeds and poppy seeds. While the former is heaty in nature, the latter is cooling and thus helps to balance the dish. The five spices, called pancha phodan, give it a unique taste and flavour.

Ingredients:

Cut all the following vegetables* to the length and shape of a finger:
½ cup raw green papaya
1 cup drumsticks (vegetable of moringa tree)
1 cup sweet potatoes
1/5 cup bitter gourd (karelā)
1 cup green beans
1 cup raw plantain (kaccā kelā)

Tadka (spicing)
2 tbsp extra virgin olive oil
1 tsp pancha phodan†
¾ tsp salt
Wet spices
1 tbsp mustard seeds
1 tbsp white poppy seeds

Garnish: 1 tbsp coconut milk

Directions:

- Soak mustard seeds and poppy seeds together for wet grinding.
- Cut all the vegetables roughly to the size and shape of a finger. Wash with water and drain.

---

* Bitter gourd or karela and plantain is a must for this preparation. Other vegetables can be substituted according to the season and what is locally available.

† 1 part mustard seeds, 1 part cumin seeds, 1 part fennel seeds, ½ part kalonji seeds, ½ part fenugreek seeds

- In a heavy wok, heat the oil and add the pancha phodan spices. Stir-fry till they crack open and a nice aroma of spices released. Add the vegetables and stir-fry for a few minutes. Leave them covered for some time. Add salt and stir-for a few moments. Cook till the vegetables roast well and turn brown.
- Blend the soaked seeds into a fine paste. Add 60 per cent of this to the cooking vegetables. Stir occasionally.
- Add two cups of boiling water and cook everything together till all the vegetables are cooked well and soaked with the mustard sauce. Turn off the flame and add the fresh coconut milk. Stir.
- Serve hot with soft hot steamed rice.

The Right Method of Serving and Eating

'The way to one's heart is through one's stomach.'

—African Proverb

It is important to do a few things before we sit down to eat. It is best that your stomach be empty and the previous meal be digested. It is good to bathe before eating, offer prayers to your gods and forefathers, make sure all the staff working with you has eaten to their satisfaction and any pets are well fed. Then, one can sit down with a free mind and eat with proper hunger. One should eat doṣa-friendly palatable sātmya food with loving family members. Palatable food that delights the mind and gladdens the tongue will confer enthusiasm and strength. Unpalatable food will act in the opposite way.

While ensuring the above good conduct, you should be conscious of the timing of your own eating. When the food is eaten after the appropriate time of hunger has lapsed, the digestive fire gets weakened due to disturbed vāta, and whatever is consumed is digested with difficulty with no further desire to eat afterwards. So, make sure you eat at the right time. It is better to have fresh ginger root with rock salt at the commencement of the meal to stimulate the digestive fire.

This also improves appetite and clears the tongue and throat. One should start eating food with predominantly sweet taste and then gradually shift to sour and finally to bitter, pungent and astringent tastes. If there are fruits like pomegranate, one should start the meal with it, excepting for bananas. It is also good to begin the meal with heavier items like roots and stems (lotus stem), but never have them after meals as they will increase indigestion and kapha. Fill half your stomach with solids and a quarter with liquids and leave quarter empty to be occupied by vāta and air elements for efficient digestion. Food that is piping hot will reduce strength, cold food will be difficult to digest and food that is too wet will lead to fatigue. The good and bad benefits of food are not accrued when eaten hastily (pitta prakṛti people tend to eat fast). Eating too slowly, as in the case of vāta prakṛti people, gradually makes the food pale, unattractive and unpalatable. One should eat moderately while chewing every morsel twenty-five to thirty times. Chewing not only brings out the taste better but ensures better digestion. Eat heavy food (grains, beans, dairy, oily food, etc.) till your hunger is half satiated, followed by light food (veggies from creepers, semi-liquid preparations like soups, salads, etc.) till you reach full satiation. Overeating causes physical laziness, a feeling of heaviness and abdominal discomfort. Eating (too) little causes loss of body tissues and one becomes lean and thin. Drinking excess water or not drinking it at all (though thirsty) during a meal disrupts metabolism of food. Drinking in the beginning weakens the digestive fire and too much water at the end of the meal leads to the generation of too much kapha. Drink sip by sip as you eat steadily as per your requirement. Never eat if you are very thirsty nor drink if you are very hungry. Drink when thirsty and eat when hungry. So, eat food skilfully prepared, avoiding all the mistakes just mentioned.

We should note here that serving deserves as much credit as cooking a good meal, no matter how perfect the cooking is. A warm serving hand makes the food tastier and takes it beyond perfection. One should be careful who's cooking and serving the food and thank them equally. The cook should also be thankful to the servers, otherwise all of his/her hard labour would be fruitless. Even if the cook makes a mistake, if the food is served with love, the person eating it is naturally forgiving. The server should also be grateful to the cook for cooking healthy and tasty food. All this happens congenially in a loving family atmosphere and needs to be maintained at all levels (ashram, home, restaurant, resort, etc.).

Serving Plates: A book called *Yogiplate* cannot end without discussing plates. The best utensils to eat on are those in gold and silver as considered by ancient texts. Gold and silver are known to increase immunity. Charaka says that the body of a person who is habituated to eating in gold plates becomes resistant to poison as much as a lotus leaf is resistant to water. Both gold and silver pots are alleviators of all three doṣas, enhance memory and are good for the eyes. However, it is not practical to use gold and silverware. If possible, try to invest in a few silver pots. Use a silver cup, for example, for drinking hot milk or water on a regular basis.

As for other pots, kansa promotes intelligence but is an aggravator of pitta doṣa. Iron is anti-inflammatory and good for people who have anaemia. A plate need not always be made of metal. We can use something as simple as a leaf from a tree. Banana leaves are easily found, environment-friendly, enhance taste, reduce pitta and vāta doṣa and are pleasing to the eye. Many other leaves, like palasha (pliers)leaves, sal tree leaves and lotus leaves are all beneficial and should be encouraged instead of plastic. Stainless steel is neutral and does not add any value to the food. Aluminium and plastic takes away some qualities from the food. Clay and some stone pots also enhance the taste. Wooden plates increase kapha, but reduce pitta and vāta doṣa. Plates made of natural materials enhance taste and help in balancing some doṣas. However, we should avoid choosing a vessel that would increase the doṣa which already exists in the food. For example, we should not serve sour food in kansa or bronze pots.

Apart from cooking and serving methods, food that is cooked with hatred will affect our body and mind negatively. When consumed continuously for a long period of time, one is bound to suffer from the after-effects of eating such food.

Also note, dry foods (mostly snacks) if mixed appropriately with fluids will be digested well. That's why bhel (a mixture of dry puffed rice with freshly chopped raw veggies) is better than just puffed rice with peanuts. Dry food potentially leads to constipation and thus weakens digestion. Also separately drinking water after a dry snack weakens the digestive system.

Conduct after Eating

After the meal, wash your mouth by swirling water in it several times. Remove food particles from the teeth. And rinse again. Wash your hands and feet (if possible) with cool (room temperature) water. This balances the excess pitta and leads to a smooth digestion. Gently walk for five minutes. Sitting/inaction immediately after eating results in obesity whereas a gentle walk increases your lifespan. Running immediately after eating can cause death. So immediately jumping into various passionate activities will reduce your lifespan. If your schedules demand, switch to a light meal. In all cases, it is explained in Ayurvedic literature that after a meal, one should remember Viashvānara (Lord of digestive fire) and sage Agastya (who has a mighty digestive power) while gently massaging the stomach with the right palm in circles.

Try to avoid sleeping immediately after meals as it will aggravate kapha and slow down the digestion. If it so happens, then to counter it, have a mild pungent (ginger and pepper) hot tea and take a smoke medication of agaru (not tobacco). You may lie in a supine posture for eight breaths, then on your right side for sixteen breaths and then on your left side for thirty-two breaths. After this, you may sleep as per your comfort (without indulging in it).

Conclusion

It is best to eat as much home-cooked food as possible. Make sure you apply the principles of Ayurvedic cooking as much as possible. Even small doses of medicine have a significant impact.

Besides, food binds people together very strongly. The same recipe cooked by different people will taste different, and the one who cooks with affection is bound to make tastier food.

Whenever I speak of this aspect in my workshops, I am reminded of the story of Naḷa and Damayanti. Naḷa was a powerful king and Damayanti was his dear queen. Naḷa was also an excellent and famous cook. His cooking was acclaimed by all the aristocrats. He was also an expert at training horses.

One day, unfortunately, Naḷa and Damayanti were separated. Their love for each other, however, did not diminish. Naḷa grew wan and thin as he struggled in life. Later, when fate brought them together, it was hard for Damayanti to recognize Naḷa though she felt it was him. So she requested some food cooked by him for her. As soon as she tasted it, she knew it was him.

This story is a reminder that each of us links certain tastes and dishes to very special memories. Even years apart, a person can recreate the magic and bring back the same memories for another person through a dish. So, start cooking at home for yourself and your loved ones. Start creating those memories together.

Sāttvic food cooked, served and eaten according to Ayurvedic principles benefits a person at three levels—body, mind and soul.

Afterword

'I choose to make the rest of my life the best of my life.'

—Louise L. Hay

The Sanskrit for eating is 'āhāra', which means all that which we take into our system for nourishment. Food is just one aspect. The air we inhale, the water we drink, the sounds we hear, the sights we see and the thoughts we entertain are all āhāra. When āhāra is pure and full of vitality, it will instill life and vigour in us. If the āhāra is impure, then it will take vitality away from us. If one type of āhāra is clean but not the other, then we are inviting sickness. For example, if food is clean but not the water, we will fall sick. Similarly, if the food is pure, but the mind is dwelling on negativities arising out of anger, envy or pride, then too we are likely to fall sick. When we think of nourishment, which is the basis of good health, we need to think of all these factors. A healthy diet is one that nourishes us at the level of the body, mind and imparts satisfaction to our inner self.

There are six essential things I want you to gather from this book to cultivate a culture of good health:

1. Understand your nature: both tridoṣa as well as triguṇa nature. This will help you understand your food profile and work profile. You will find your answer to this in Section One.
2. Understand the nature of the food: again both in terms of tridoṣa and triguṇa. Try to consume as much fresh and sāttvic food as possible and choose only the food that matches your tridoṣa profile.
3. Understand the strength of your digestive fire and eat accordingly. For even if the tridoṣa of food matches your tridoṣa nature, but your digestive fire is not ready, you will suffer from undigested food which creates āma or toxins in the body. It's also important to learn which food and tastes (rasa) are good for you and are digested smoothly and which are not. Which food suits you in a particular season and which does not and the quantity of food you should be eating for a particular meal. Take into account details of imbalances in particular doṣas (due to jetlag, late-night work to finish a project, etc.). All these factors influence our digestion. In any case, wait for hunger to arise before eating your meal.

If there is an imbalance in the doṣa, first address that issue. For example, if you are experiencing bloating and gas owing to imbalance in the vāta doṣa, then sip a cup of hot water or hot water with less than a quarter teaspoon of ajwain (carom) seeds to subdue it. If pitta is high, drink cool water or water with misri and soaked dry kokam (mangosteen or garcinia indica) fruit. If kapha is high, then have a cup of hot ginger jaggery tea (kadha) to soothe the cough and ignite the digestive fire. In this way, find the means to pacify your imbalanced doṣas and then wait for the hunger. Eat according to the level of hunger. Once you are well nourished, your body will gradually return to its normal level of hunger over a period of time.

4. Include a good exercise plan that suits your nature because good exercise will keep the digestive fire tidy and free the mind from stress. Walking, jogging, trekking, bicycling, outdoor sports, any of these or a combination of all of these would be best. Yoga is universal to all. The specialty of yoga is it takes care of intricate organs like pancreas, thyroid glands etc., in a very effective way. In that sense Yoga is indispensable. We have discussed a specific yoga procedure, called agnisāra kriyā, to ignite the digestive fire. Try applying it in your exercise routine.
5. Take out time to relax your mind. Relaxation, especially in this age and time, is the key to good digestive fire. A mentally exhausted person cannot digest food well. Good sleep and meditation are essential here. Whereas sleep is a state in which we forget everything, meditation helps one go inward and transcend the effects of stress.

   We have discussed how stress seizes the digestive system. Even if we have understood our nature and eat food suiting our tridoṣa nature, we may not be able to digest it if stressed. The Bhagavad Gitā advises one to perform work in a spirit of sacrifice to stay immune to stress (*yajñārthāt karmaṇo 'nyatra BG 3.9*).
6. Finally, learn the art of combining food ingredients to cook a perfect meal following the rules of Dinacaryā and Ṛtucaryā. When you cook your own food, in the back of your mind, you are aware about your doṣa constitution and doṣa imbalances, and these will be naturally incorporated.

Or if someone else is cooking for you, you should let them know about your diet. This is mindful cooking. Of course, mindful cooking also includes the care, concern and affection one feels while cooking with a spirit of sacrifice. The best food comes from the hands of that cook who maintains a spirit of sacrifice and the motive is not to enjoy the food he/she cooks, rather to nourish the people who are eating.

Also make sure to stay away from processed food that contains many chemicals. Even if the potatoes used in making a bag of chips are organic and the oil for frying is good, there are so many other steps, like washing the potatoes, that might involve chemicals. Also, the mindfulness of the cook is generally far less in such products.

When you understand the above six principles (Chart 6.1) and apply them in your life you will relish a healthy life at the level of body, mind and inner self. The impact of imbalanced doṣas is destructive and causes diseases. To thrive is a constant struggle. It's not always possible to avoid disease. It is best to remain cautious about your diet and health, and try to find your way back in case you get derailed. Staying humble and living life as an example to serve will keep us happy.

Although I have tried to cover different categories of food ingredients (grains, vegetables, dairy, oil etc.) many are still missing in this book. The idea was to discuss the principles and quote examples that have been tried and tested. So I request you to gather these principles and utilize them to benefit you considering the time, place and circumstances. Looking forward, be aware of your body,

Chart 6.1: Questions to Ask before Eating

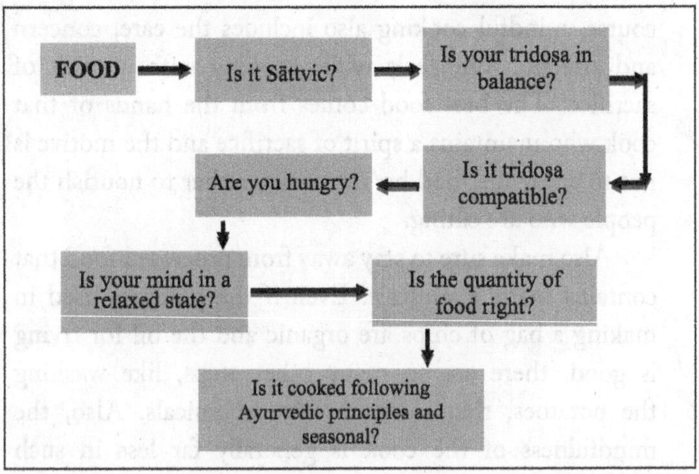

mind and the surrounding and decide the course of action. It is no rocket science, but mere awareness and sincere practice. Life is precious. My best wishes to each of you for a happy and healthy life.

Acknowledgements

I humbly thank my spiritual master, His Holiness Radhanath Swami, whose loving blessings and kind appreciations inspired me to dig deep into culinary culture. I thank Dr Sanjay Pisharodi who was instrumental in inspiring and convincing me that this book is indeed the need of the hour. Unfortunately, he left us in a road accident before I could even start writing this book. I am ever grateful to him.

Sincere thanks to my mentors, Vaisesika Dasa Adhikari, Gauranga Das and Govind Das for inspiring me in all my welfare activities. Gauranga Das, who happily agreed to write a foreword to this book, has been my guide and a friend since the mid-1990s. He recognized the chef in me and opened up massive opportunities that kept me busy beyond my expectations. He also cooked along with me to serve millions. This book is actually a result of all those intense actions which I call: the culinary craze.

I thank Radhakunda Das, a dear friend who inspired me to take up a Yoga Teacher's Training programme. I also thank Robert Sankara Moses and Swami Govindananda Saraswati for awarding the yoga and prāṇāyāma training and deepening my understanding of yoga and sāttvic diet. I thank Rajeev Pandita, who tirelessly helped me to teach the science and skills of sāttvic cooking.

I thank my family at Bhubaneswar, my roots: including my elder sister Smrutirekha and her husband Rashmiranjan, Richie and Rishu (my niece and nephew) and Smarajeet, my elder brother. Each of them shaped me up in innumerable ways. I am always grateful to them. My sincere gratitude to my mother and father, whose simple sāttvic cooking and their own examples helped me face all adversities in my life without losing hope and harming anybody.

Penguin Random House India approached me to write this book soon after Hansapriya, my dear wife, entered my life. She provided me with all the support and space I needed to write this book. She inspired me constantly and thought the book would be a wonderful source of helpful information for one and all. I can't thank her enough. My father-in-law, who has brought prostate cancer under full control at the age of seventy-six, just by following specific diet plans, fasting and some yogic kriyās, has been an amazing source of inspiration, and has filled the void of my father, who left us a decade back.

I thank innumerable wonderful cooks, working in their homes, Vedic temples, monasteries, restaurants, roadside shops, guesthouses, etc. who happily shared their secrets.

I thank Dr S.K.C. Prabhu and Dr Ruchira N. Garodia for preventing possible errors while describing the Ayurvedic principles. They guided and inspired me throughout the writing. My sincere heartfelt thanks to them. The book evolved well because of their constant inputs and inspirations.

I also thank many websites featuring useful articles that I studied and referred to for this writing. Notably, I truly appreciate Dr J.V. Hebbar, who has put a wealth of information on easyayurveda.com.

My sincere thanks to Roshini Dadlani, Associate Commissioning Editor at Penguin, for editing the book. Her interest in this project and her practising the Ayurvedic principles as she edited the book was quite fulfilling. She asked all possible questions that a reader would probably look for and made the writing a smooth presentation for all. Indeed, I thank the entire publishing team, notably Saloni Mital and Nicholas Rixon for bringing this book to all of you smoothly. It was a great pleasure working with them all. Also, my sincere thanks to Devangana Dash for designing the cover page, various artworks and publishing the book. I thank Sandesh Borgaonkar, a friend and brother, who happily agreed to do the photography for the cover page. My sincere thanks to Dr Chaitanya Polla for proofreading and providing valuable inputs.

I thank Bhaktivedanta Swami Prabhupada, a personality who has inspired me intensely in my spiritual journey, for rendering the Bhagavad Gitā into English as it is. I referred to his translations while defining sāttvic food.

Finally my obeisance with all humility to Dhanawantri, the Lord of Ayurveda and specially to Sri Sri Radha Gopinathji, my sole object of worship.